I0650000

WILLIAM COOKWORTHY

WILLIAM COOKWORTHY
1705 - 1780

A STUDY OF THE PIONEER OF TRUE
PORCELAIN MANUFACTURE IN ENGLAND

JOHN PENDERILL–CHURCH

BRADFORD BARTON
TRURO

first published 1972 *by*
D. BRADFORD BARTON LIMITED
TRETHELLAN HOUSE · TRURO · CORNWALL
printed in Great Britain by
H. E. WARNE LIMITED · ST. AUSTELL

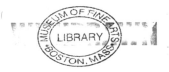

CONTENTS

ILLUSTRATIONS

PREFACE

IT HAS BEEN SAID THAT THE FATE OF ALL DISCOVERERS
and inventors is to be forgotten, whilst their discoveries and
inventions become known the world over. This is true of the
discoverers of bacteria, electricity, oxygen, penicillin and vitamins
and also true of the inventors of steam propulsion, the telephone,
television and the jet propulsion engine. It is equally true of the
discoverer of china clay in Cornwall and the inventor of the first
British process for the manufacture of hard paste porcelain. The
man who both discovered the clay and invented a process to make
use of it, was the Quaker chemist, William Cookworthy. In the
following pages it is my aim to present as clear as possible a
picture of this extraordinary man, who crammed more into his
seventy-five year lifetime than any two or three other men put
together.

William Cookworthy has, in the past, been described as "the
man whose biography can never be written". This is due to the
fact that historians are very much at variance with each other as to
when he did this and that, where he did it, indeed if he did it at all.
In fact, there are only two facts concerning him that have not
been disputed—one, that he was born, and two, that he died!
Various authorities cannot even agree on the date of his death,
some saying October 16th and others October 17th. There has
even been disagreement in the past about the number of daughters
he had, different accounts crediting him with four, five and seven.
Much of the trouble in establishing an accurate account of his
life has been due to the fact that his three principal biographers,
although all related or descended from him, never actually set
eyes on him, but received such information as they had about him
secondhand, from mothers, grandmothers and the like. George
Harrison, for instance, was the son of Susanna Harrison *nee*
Cookworthy, the chemist's youngest daughter. He was not born
until 1790, ten years after Cookworthy's death. His mother, who
was his principal source of information, died when he was only

20 years old, and after that he was only able to pick up scraps of information here and there. Theodore Compton married Elizabeth Harrison, daughter of the above mentioned George Harrison and such information as he had was very much at second-, or even third-hand. John Prideaux, the main source of general knowledge concerning Cookworthy, was the great-grandson of Philip Cookworthy, William's second youngest brother whose daughter Anna had married George Prideaux. Prideaux had another source of information other than his own mother, as his wife was a Nancarrow, great grand-daughter of Cookworthy's great friend, John Nancarrow, senior mine captain of the Godolphin group of mines, including Great Work and Wheal Grey, in whose workings Cookworthy first discovered china clay.

With the three main biographers all relying on what had been passed on by word of mouth, it is quite understandable that the accounts vary considerably. To produce a one-hundred per cent accurate biography was not possible then and is not even possible now. Fortunately, however, various gaps in our information concerning Cookworthy have been filled in from a number of different sources, so that it has now become possible to present a fuller picture of the man and his work. Cookworthy's contribution to the world is perhaps greater than most people would realise. China clay, although still used for ceramic purposes in potteries all over the world, is even more widely used in the paper industry, both as a filler and a coating agent. More than 75 per cent of all china clay produced is destined for use in the paper trade, whilst only 15 per cent or thereabouts is destined for use in ceramics. The remainder is divided between rubber, paint, fertilizers, insecticides and pharmaceutical applications. No doubt, china clay would have been exploited in Cornwall eventually, even without Cookworthy, but when?—that is a question no-one can answer. Long after Cookworthy's excursions to Tregonning Hill, 84 years to be precise, the first china clay was discovered at Lee Moor—although Cookworthy had seen occurrences of poor quality clay not far away, either at Hemerdon or Redlake. It was not until about 1850, over one hundred years after both Tregonning and St. Stephen's clays had been discovered, that china clay was first discovered on Bodmin Moor, or

perhaps rediscovered is a better word, since Trehawke first
spotted it around 1755.

There have been in the past various persons who have en-
deavoured to belittle Cookworthy's achievements, claiming that
the real honour of starting the china clay industry should go to
Josiah Wedgwood and John Turner of Lane End, who opened up
clay country to the Staffordshire pottery industry as a whole in
1775 by contesting Richard Champion's application for a
renewal of the Cookworthy patent. The fact remains, however,
that neither Wedgwood nor Turner would have recognised a
lump of china clay if they had seen it. Without Cookworthy's
insight and intuition, they would never have known of its
existence. Wedgwood himself, whilst accompanying his brother
Dr. Thomas Wedgwood as his agent, actually handled china
clay from Tregonning Hill in 1749, when he was nineteen years
of age, but never recognised it for what it was. He was later given
a sample of American china clay from Cherokee country in
South Carolina, but again would not have recognised what it was
if he had not been told previously. He was a potter, not a chemist,
even though he had scientific leanings.

Other members of the anti-Cookworthy faction have pointed
out that the Cornish already knew of the existence of china clay
long before William Cookworthy. This is true. They knew that
the whitish substance which they called pot growan, pry wyn, or
fluccan, when made into a stiff paste, moulded into rectangular
blocks and fired, produced excellent refractory bricks for use in
the hearths of steam pumping engines as well as the fireplaces in
the tin smelting houses. They also knew that it could be used to
produce crucibles, but what they did not know was that this
substance, so ordinary and commonplace in their estimation, was
the same as the Kaolin referred to by Du Halde, and could be
used to manufacture porcelain. It took Cookworthy to deduce
that pot growan and kaolin were one and the same, and that
moorstone in its semi-decomposed form was identical with
petuntse.

Although it is with his work on china clay that Cookworthy
is usually associated, in the minds of the few who remember his
existence, the finding and utilisation of china clay was only a
fraction of his total work. Before even James Lynd had announced

his discovery of an anti-scorbutic factor in fresh vegetables and fruits in 1759, Cookworthy already knew that it was lack of vegetables on long voyages which produced scurvy, and had recommended that fresh vegetables should be supplemented on board ship with sauerkraut, and before even Koch had isolated his first bacteria, Cookworthy already knew that there was some factor present in foul water that was not present in fresh water, and which, where present, was the cause of diseases. It was for this reason that he devised a method of distilling sea water on board ships, so that really fresh water could be always available.

Cookworthy himself regarded his work with clays to be of very minor importance, compared with his work as a Quaker Minister. He thought that his most important calling was to preach the word of God to members of the Society of Friends wherever and whenever possible, and to be a saver of souls when there were souls to be saved. With the exception of his article on the use of the divining rod, his method for distilling water, the 1765 memorandum and the 1768 patent, and a few odd letters, his entire literary output consisted of counsels on the spiritual life, dissertations on various matters, exhortations to the faithful and notes of his various spiritual experiences when journeying around the country as a Quaker minister. This may make him sound as if he was a religious bore, but he was not. He was capable of talking at length on any subject that people liked to mention, and not merely to talk, but to make intelligent and apposite observations on that subject. As a conversationalist, he made friends with many clever men—Sir Joseph Banks, Captain Cook, Captain Jervis, Dr. Mudge, Sir Joshua Reynolds, John Smeaton, Dr. Daniel Solander, Dr. Emmanuel Swedenborg and Dr. John Wolcot (otherwise known as the satirist Peter Pindar). None of these were the sort of man that suffers fools gladly, and each and everyone of them knew very well that Cookworthy was no fool.

With such exalted friends, it might be thought that Cookworthy was an intellectual snob, but the opposite was the case. He would hold a conversation with anyone from a peer to a ploughman, and in spite of all his rich and influential customers at the Notte Street pharmacy, he never neglected his poorer customers, many of whom could not afford to pay him except in kind. That he was universally loved and admired in Plymouth can be borne out by the fact that when he died, not only the Quakers, but people from all walks of life, rich and poor alike, dropped what they were doing and followed the coffin in procession from Notte Street to the Friends Meeting House, which was so full that some people could not get in at all, and were forced to listen to the service through the open doors.

Such then, was the man William Cookworthy—Quaker Minister, apothecary, conversationalist, philanthropist, ceramist, artist, all combined into one, as one of the extraordinary characters produced by the eighteenth century; a man of many parts, all of them good, a Jack of many trades, of each of which he was a master.

I. BIRTH TO MANHOOD

IN 1704, A PROSPEROUS WEAVER, WILLIAM COOKWORTHY, living and working at Kingsbridge in South Devon, married a Cornish girl, Edith Debell, daughter of John and Mary Debell of St. Martin's by Looe. He was a weaver of woollen materials and member of the Guild of Weavers, but above all else, he was a member of the Society of Friends, or as it is more commonly put, a Quaker. His wife was also a Quaker, from the community of Friends at Looe. Whilst most people at that time married other people from their own or neighbouring villages, the Quakers had already abolished the parochial outlook amongst their followers, so that there was no fuss made about William's marrying someone from so far away as Looe. Some four months after their marriage, Edith Cookworthy became pregnant, and in due course was delivered of a son, on April 12th 1705. This son was named William after his father. He was destined to be remembered, long after his parents had been forgotten, as a man by whose insight a great industry was able to come into being, namely the china clay industry.

In the ensuing years, William and Edith were to have six more children—Sarah born in 1706, Jacob born in 1709, Susanna born in 1711, Mary born in 1714, Philip in 1716 and the last of their children, Benjamin, born in 1718. Young William, from the time that he could walk, showed an extraordinary interest in everything around him. His parents could see that here was a child of unusual intelligence, but deliberately avoided letting him know it, so that he should not grow up conceited in any way. In 1710, young William started his first schooling at Kingsbridge. From the very beginning, he showed an unusual aptitude for learning, picking up the alphabet straight away, and becoming able to read when still very young. His teacher, realising the true calibre of this pupil, even at such an early age, discussed his academic future with his parents. It was tentatively agreed that he would be taken as far as he could go educationally at Kingsbridge

School, and would then be transferred to another school to complete his learning, possibly finishing off at a University if his brilliance at study continued to last.

In 1711, the year that Susanna was born, the South Sea Company was floated, and many people invested large sums of money in it, some entrusting nearly all their life's savings. It was, however, a doubtful concern, and that able and shrewd politician, Sir Robert Walpole, instinctively distrusted it from the onset, not being afraid to say so in public and risk unpopularity. In spite of Walpole's gloomy prognostications, the shares attracted the public's notice, and began a boom on the Stock Market. Amongst those who bought shares was William Cookworthy senior. He invested nearly all of his life savings in the Company apart from such financial interests as he had in other Quaker business undertakings. He was no fool, normally, in business matters, but greater men than him were to succumb to temptation and purchase shares in the Company before it finally collapsed. For the first few years everything looked promising, and apparently assured of future prosperity, William and Edith had more children. Meanwhile, young William continued his schooling, proving to have a natural ability to learn languages, acquiring Latin and Greek with much greater ease than his fellows. He was not entirely a bookworm, however, being interested in everything around him—the local industries such as agriculture, weaving, woodwork and fishing, even taking an interest in the local blacksmith's work and the work of a local pottery producing the well known South Devon red "cloam" or earthenware. The art of the potter interested him particularly, and if he had been allowed, would have stood watching the potter at work with his wheel for hours. Later in life he was to compare God's shaping the purpose of mankind to the potter shaping the soft clay on his humble wheel. Apart from his interest in local industry, he was also interested in nature, loving to walk in the still unspoilt countryside along Devon's leafy lanes, learning the names of the flowers and the wild birds he encountered. From his elders, he learnt the medicinal uses of the more common herbs amongst the plants he saw, because at that time most housewives still relied to a large extent on herbal medicine for their more minor ailments.

When he was old enough, William was transferred to another school at Exeter, but he was not destined to remain there for very long. In 1718, Benjamin, William's youngest brother, was born. Although his parents were not to know it, his destiny, together with that of his brother Philip, was to be closely tied to that of their eldest brother. On October 22nd, tragedy struck the Cookworthy household for the first time, when William Cookworthy Senior died. He was of no great age, and would have been forty-eight if he had lived another few weeks until his birthday, November 8th. The full repercussions of his death were not felt immediately, as there was still some income from the shares in the South Sea Company and from his other business interests. Fortunately, Edith Cookworthy was a very capable and practical woman, used to managing on a small income as a result of her experiences during her Cornish childhood, and so she managed to make ends meet, by taking in needlework, with the help she received from other members of the Society of Friends in the neighbourhood. In 1720, however, another disaster befell the family, when the South Sea Company collapsed. This happening was called, at the time, "the bursting of the South Sea Bubble", and through its collapse, a great number of people, including the Cookworthys, were financially ruined.

Up to this time, William had been able, by means of scholarships, to remain at school, but now, at the age of fifteen, it was his duty to support the family. It was no longer possible for him to contemplate a University career. Both he and Jacob had to obtain employment locally to help make ends meet, with five younger children's mouths to fill. It was at this juncture that Fate, which had hitherto dealt so unkindly with the Cookworthy family, gave them a helping hand. Five years previously, in 1715, two Welsh Quaker apothecaries, Timothy and Sylvanus Bevan of Swansea, had come to London and established there a pharmacy at Plough Court. This Plough Court Pharmacy had prospered, and the two brothers were now quite comfortably off. Apart from their pharmaceutical activities, the brothers were both preachers, and travelled the countryside visiting various Quaker communities and preaching to them. During 1720 one of the brothers visited the community at Kingsbridge, and during his stay was acquainted with the plight of the Cookworthy family. He called on Edith Cookworthy at her home, and there met her eldest son William. Bevan was immediately drawn towards this keen intelligent boy, and enquired what he intended to make his profession. When William told him, Bevan immediately realised what a waste of such obvious talent this would be. He asked William if he knew Latin and Greek, and William told him that he had been learning both these languages up to the time of the death of his father. Bevan then asked if he knew anything about medicine, and William told him what he knew concerning the medicinal uses of various herbs and mineral salts. By now, Bevan was very impressed, and suggested to Edith Cookworthy that he should take William on as an apprentice at the Plough Court Pharmacy. Mrs. Cookworthy said that she would have been only too willing for her son to be apprenticed had her circumstances allowed, but that she was afraid it would be necessary to refuse his offer because she could not afford the apprenticeship fees. Bevan straight away said that he would waive the question of fees, provided that William would live in with the Bevans and make himself generally useful in the household.

When William heard the news of the opportunity which had been offered him, he was overjoyed, but one thing concerned him—how to get to London in the first place. If he were to ride there, he would need a good horse, because the way was long and the road uneven, but a horse was something he did not possess and could not afford to buy. He could have taken the stage-coach either from Plymouth or Exeter, but that also was out of the question because of the cost. Thinking it over, he decided that as he was fifteen and physically fit, although thin and wiry in build, he would *walk* to London. This was no mean undertaking, and at first Mrs. Cookworthy would not hear of it, but seeing the look of determination in the eye of her first born, she realised that if anyone could accomplish such a trip, he would be that one. He got together his few meagre possessions into a bundle, and selected his strongest most weatherproof coat and stoutest shoes for the journey. Taking what little money his mother could spare for food and accommodation on the way, and equipping himself with a strong staff to support him and ward off any possible attack by footpads he duly set out. As he waved goodbye to the family, there was not a dry eye in the household, and even he shed a secret tear at the thought of leaving his family, although reassuring himself with the thought "What God wills, I will".

Whether he realised that the distance he would have to cover was, in fact, 240 miles, is not known, but he must have known that he had a long way to go, and yet his heart did not fail him. He is believed to have gone via Totnes, Exeter, Taunton, Westbury, Newbury and Reading. The roads must have seemed very long and very lonely in between each town, and many a lesser person would have been too frightened to walk along some stretches. This was the era not only of footpads but also of highwaymen. When he was asked afterwards whether he had not been afraid of encountering either of these species of rogues, he replied "There was nought for them to take from me, save my life, and that is of little value". The most lonely parts of his great walk must have been those parts where he skirted Salisbury Plain and crossed the Berkshire Downs. Here, he would have seen very few living souls, but seen many remains of prehistoric man, and may have pondered on the immensity of God's time compared with the short flung lives of men. Having very little money, *en route* he sought out the houses of fellow Quakers wherever possible. There were quite strong communities of Quakers in towns like Exeter, Taunton and Reading. In spite of the rough road surfaces, the roads being rutty or stony, or at times little better than muddy tracks, he averaged thirty-two miles a day, which was good going for a grown man, let alone a fifteen year old.

Eventually, weary, dusty and travel-stained, he reached the outskirts of London and saw the towers and spires of the city looming through the mist. He asked his way to Plough Court, and after being misdirected several times and having to endure ribbing from the Cockneys because of his soft Devonshire burr, he finally arrived on the Bevans' doorstep. When he knocked on the door, Mrs. Bevan opened it. Seeing such a bedraggled figure, she thought for a moment that he was a beggar, and was going to close the door in his face, but boldened by necessity, he asked her if this was the house of Timothy and Sylvanus Bevan. She replied that it was, but with true Welsh caution, still would not let him in, until he explained that he was William Cookworthy, and that Mr. Bevan had agreed to take him on as an apprentice. As soon as she heard who he was, her heart went out to the fatherless boy, and she took him in. Within a short while she had warm water to wash his blistered feet, a warm drink and a bite to eat ready for him. When he had rested, she showed him to his room in the attic, very small and cramped, but being in the roof, he could get a little more air than if he had been on the ground floor.

For the next five years he lived with the Bevans and shared their family life and family worship. All this time he was very poor, and had but the one camlet coat to his back, the same one which he had worn on his long walk. He received good wholesome food, however, and the Bevans lent him a great many books so that he could further his education. It was a hard life for a boy of his age. The Plough Court Pharmacy was fashionable, and he had to run many errands to the homes of the wealthy. In addition he had to keep the pharmacy clean, and clean up all the pestles and mortars, mixing jars and other equipment in use at the pharmacy, as well as grinding down gums and resins, crushing roots and preparing ointments for use in the pharmacy. He was kept at work from first light in the morning until it got dark. When he finally retired to his little attic he would take with him a stump of candle or a cheap tallow dip, and would sit long into the night studying for all he was worth. He studied many subjects—*materia medica*, therapeutics, Latin, Greek, chemistry and physics. He even found time to learn French, although how he did it remains a mystery. All his learning was eventually to stand him in very good stead.

During the five years of his apprenticeship, Timothy and Sylvanus Bevan found that their initial appraisal of his worth was fully justified. His brain was like a dry sponge, ready to absorb every drop of knowledge it could find. He had the valuable ability of remembering things, even when he had only been told them the once. By the end of the apprenticeship, the brothers could see that by dint of asking, searching and reading, he had acquired a knowledge of materia medica as good as their own, and they had been in the pharmaceutical business for many years longer than he had. He proved to be very skilful in mixing and compounding drugs, preparing tinctures, mixtures and draughts and making pills and cachets. His skill at mixing was to stand him in good stead in later years, when he faced the task of mixing the necessary ingredients in order to manufacture porcelain. Eventually the day came when his apprenticeship was finally over and he emerged as a fully fledged apothecary.

He was now twenty years old, but in many ways he was old for his years. He could hold an intelligent conversation with men many years his elder, and was never at a loss for words. His eloquence led the Bevans to believe that he would make a valuable preacher to the Society of Friends, as in fact he did, serving the Quaker cause faithfully right up to the time of his death. Being now qualified, the Bevan brothers considered what should be his future. They did not want to lose so apt a pupil altogether, and so they offered him a partnership in the firm. William would have gladly accepted this, but he was worrying about how his mother was coping with things in Kingsbridge. Jacob was out at work, it was true, but that still left the other mouths to feed. Realising his concern for his family, the Bevans hit on another idea. Plymouth was then becoming a very important place, due to its rise as a naval port. They had already considered expanding their interests to places other than London and Swansea, and what better place for a new venture than Plymouth? So it was that a new pharmacy was opened up in Notte Street on the site of the present Elim Church. It was called Bevan and Cookworthy, Dispensing Chemists, and its manager, at the age of 20, was William Cookworthy.

II. THE YOUNG APOTHECARY

THE NOTTE STREET PHARMACY WAS A SUCCESS FROM the start. To begin with, Cookworthy managed largely on his own, except for a boy to run errands and do chores for him. News of his skill as an apothecary spread quickly around the town, and he began to attract a great number of customers, poor and rich alike, including a number of Naval officers. It was through his Naval contacts that he was able to secure the contract for the supply of drugs to the ships putting into Plymouth, a contract which was to assure him of a steady trade for the whole of his lifetime and to continue through the lives of his descendants. Plymouth at that time was quite important as a commercial port, as well as a Naval port. Cookworthy soon found himself serving the captains and crew of merchantmen, as well as of Naval vessels. Considering the very limited knowledge of medicine possessed at that time even by the very best physicians, Cookworthy was quite successful in treating the more common ailments. He had a natural gift of intuition into the possible causes of diseases, even if there were no drugs available at the time to treat them. One disease which greatly affected the crews of Naval vessels and merchantmen alike was scurvy. Cookworthy was one of the earliest men to recognise that it could be caused by lack of fresh vegetables, or fruit of any sort during the later stages of voyages. He was quick to observe, on hearing the reports of ships' physicians, that the disease did not come on directly after they had been in port, while stocks of vegetables lasted, but only after they had been many weeks at sea, and it was his idea that the ships should carry casks of sauerkraut, pickled cabbage, to supplement the fresh vegetables during long voyages.

Another disease which troubled seamen was Foulwater Fever. This was known to be brought on by drinking "fresh" water that had ceased to be fresh. Carrying fresh water was always a problem. Cookworthy, however, was not to hit on a solution to the problem at this time, but like every other affliction of mankind, it concerned him. He was the sort of man that would not easily give up a struggle to find the answer to life's problems. One facet of his character which earned him many friends outside Quaker circles was his concern. If people were ill it concerned him, and he immediately became involved. If people were in trouble, he was concerned also. With him, where science left off, sympathy began. People were always assured of a patient hearing and wise advice.

Shortly after the opening of the Notte Street Pharmacy, Cookworthy's younger brother Philip decided to seek his fortune as ship's boy on board an East Indiaman—a fast sailing clipper plying to and from China and the Dutch East Indies. Edith Cookworthy did not like the idea of her son going to sea, and William Cookworthy, knowing only too well what sort of conditions his brother was likely to encounter, sought to persuade him to change his mind, but without result. William gave Philip such advice as he could as to how to keep healthy on the long voyages, and provided him with some simple medicines in case of sickness. Philip was not the most robust of boys, and his brother wondered how he would cope, but thought that it would either make or mar him. Nevertheless, as he told Philip before his first departure "If God wills, you will, so be of good heart, and trust in Him."

During the next few years Philip made a number of journeys to and from the Far East. They were not comfortable journeys by any manner of means—sometimes he would have to endure howling gales and lashing rains, whilst at other times the ship might be becalmed for days on end in shark-infested seas, with the sharks circling round all the time waiting for anything which might come their way. On the return journeys he brought gifts for the family including some true oriental porcelain for his brother—thus it was that William for the first time beheld the material he was later destined to try so hard to produce. Philip, unfortunately, knew nothing of the methods of its manufacture, only knowing that it was made up in the hills and subsequently brought down to the coast to be exported. No doubt William was curious as to its composition, as was everyone else at that time. Bottger, of course was already producing porcelain in Saxony, but his process and the materials he used remained closely guarded secrets, under the instructions of Friedrich Augustus, Elector of Saxony. In any case, the German porcelain, although hard paste like that of the Chinese, was not exactly identical to it.

Apart from all his other activities, Cookworthy was a vigorously practising Quaker, and even this time, when not yet twenty-five years old, he was a convinced and convincing preacher. He began to preach the word of God not only to the people of Plymouth, but also to the people living further afield. By this time he had purchased his first horse, a grey mare called Prudence, according to tradition, and this faithful beast was destined to carry him for many miles into many strange places ere she was too old to be of further use. From Plymouth he would journey out to Plympton, Plymstock, and Ivybridge, or to the South Hams, South Brent, Yelverton, Buckland, Tamerton Foliot and Bere Alston. As he went, he would make keen observations of all he saw, the wild plants, the birds and the animals and the condition of the people. He found a great and true peace on his long rides which he referred to as his "communion with God and with nature". No matter how physically wearying his long rides to and from preaching engagements were, he always returned spiritually refreshed and with a renewed enthusiasm for the spiritual life.

In 1729, when Philip returned from one of his long voyages, Cookworthy could see that he had had a rough time. Enquiries from his shipmates revealed that he had been sick during a great part of the voyage, although he himself would not admit to having been ill. Edith Cookworthy, with a mother's unerring instinct, had felt during the voyage that all was not well with her Philip, and when she finally saw him, her worst fears were confirmed. She once again asked William if he could prevail upon Philip to give up the sea, as he was obviously not suited to a seafaring life. Going round the coasts from port to port in a sailing barque was one thing, but travelling through strange seas for thousands of miles, sometimes with weeks or even months between putting into port was another. Mrs. Cookworthy was convinced that if Philip continued to go to sea, he would end up in an early and watery grave. Philip, however, was still obdurate, and continued to stick to his chosen trade, hard though it must have been for him to do so.

By 1730, the Notte Street Pharmacy was doing so well, that Cookworthy thought that he could justifiably take on an apprentice, one who might later become a partner. So it was, that on Philip's return from a particularly unpleasant voyage, during which he had been racked with fever, when Cookworthy offered him an apprenticeship, he took it. He was then only fifteen years of age, but his experiences at sea, coupled with the rough companionship of his messmates, had aged him, so that he could have passed for older, eighteen or nineteen at least. He was still no more robust than when he had started, being rather lean and wiry of build, the same as his eldest brother. Philip proved to have a quick mind, like his brother, and absorbed all the knowledge that William could give him. He had already been familiar with some of the more common medicaments as a result of his experience on board ship, so that the task of learning his trade did not come so hard to him as it would to one without any previous training. Within three years, he was competent enough to be able to execute the less elaborate tasks and to make up the medicaments most frequently in use. In 1733, Cookworthy's youngest brother, Benjamin, was also taken on as an apprentice, and proved that even if he was the youngest of the Cookworthys, he was no whit less endowed with brains. The pharmacy, by now, was becoming a real family concern, and the thought of it gave Edith Cookworthy a deep and lasting pleasure. Only one thing bothered her—she did wish that Cookworthy would get himself a wife. He was twenty eight years of age, but looked older, because of his early maturity. It was true that people married older in those days, but over a certain age marriages became progressively rarer.

From 1733, with two brothers involved in the business, Cookworthy was able to venture a little farther afield with medical supplies. As he went, he always made careful mental notes of all he saw, and was continually on the lookout for strange and unusual minerals. It was at this time that he began to journey into Cornwall, visiting his Debell cousins at Looe, and covering many miles of rough moorland track on his faithful mare. It is said to have been 1733 or thereabouts when he first made the acquaintance of Daniel Gumb. Today, this character has assumed an almost legendary nature, but in the beginning he was solid flesh and blood. Daniel was a stone-mason by profession, and at an early age he was left parentless. He became more and more solitary by nature, year by year, until he at last left his village and went to live up in the bleak high hills between Caradon and Tregarrick Tor. He eventually built himself a house out of the natural rocks of the hillside near the Cheesewring, and there it was, on a visit to Minions, that Cookworthy met him for the first time. Daniel was in his way something of a philosopher, as was Cookworthy, and in the following years this strangely assorted pair became firm friends.

It was during the 1730's, according to tradition, that Cookworthy saw china clay for the first time. This was at a bell foundry in Fowey. The casting of bells was prone to give rise from time to time to an industrial disease known as bellfounders' ague, the symptoms of which disease including sweating, shivering and internal cramps. The metal of which the bells were cast consisted of an alloy known as bell metal, made up usually of three to four parts of copper to one of tin and a little lead or zinc. Whilst visiting the foundry in a professional capacity, to supply such drugs as were available for the treatment of this ague, Cookworthy went actually into the casting shop to see for himself the conditions under which bells were cast. It was there that he saw a whitish powdery material being used to prepare moulds for casting. This powder, when fired had something of the appearance of unglazed porcelain. Cookworthy's interest was immediately aroused. "Tell me, pray," he said to the founder-master, "what is the white stuff of which you are making these moulds?" "Why," replied the founder-master, "'tis but the pot growan that comes from up yonder somewhere in the hills. 'Tis what we always use, and our fathers used it afore us." If only Du Halde had published his paper, Cookworthy would have probably realised what this white substance was, but as it was, he merely made a mental note of what it was called before going on his way.

In 1735, Cookworthy, doing quite well for himself by this time, married a Quakeress from Somerset, Sarah Berry, originally hailing from Wellington but living at Taunton. Sarah's family were associated with the woollen weaving industry, as Cookworthy's father had been. Her sister was married to Thomas

Were of Wellington, who manufactured woollen goods out of
the cloth woven by the Berrys. Sarah was to bear Cookworthy
five children before her untimely and early death. Edith Cookworthy was relieved to see her eldest son happily married, as she
was then sixty four, and had been wondering whether she would
live long enough to see and enjoy some grand-children. As it
happened, she was destined to outlive her daughter-in-law, dying
at the ripe old age of 88.

In 1736, Cookworthy's first daughter Lydia was born. Although he did not know it, he was destined to be inflicted with
"the Curse of Cornwall"—all female children. The same year
saw the publication in France of an important paper. This was
Du Halde's "A Description of the Empire of China and of
Chinese Tartary".

This may not sound particularly significant, merely judging by
the title, but what was so important about this paper was that it
contained details of the materials used and the method of manufacture of hard porcelain in China. These details had been
originally sent by a Jesuit Father, Pere d'Entrecolles, to a friend of
his, the Baron de Reaumur, together with samples of the raw
materials. D'Entrecolles had seen the materials whilst he was
engaged in missionary work at King-te-Ching and had, by dint
of patient questioning, elicited the fact that they were the materials
used in the making of porcelain. It is not known whether Cookworthy read Du Halde's paper in the original French, or whether
in fact he read Richard Brooke's translation which was produced
in the following year, although it did not become generally
available until several years later. Whichever was the case, he
certainly read, learnt and inwardly digested the contents in no
uncertain manner, and mentally resolved that he would find the
same materials in the West Country, if they were in fact there to
be found.

During the next few years, Cookworthy did not spend quite
so much time travelling abroad as he had done prior to his
marriage. Sarah was busy bearing him children—the next after
Lydia being Sarah, born in 1738, followed by Mary in 1740 and
the twins, Elizabeth and Susanna born in 1743. Having the twins
rather debilitated Sarah, and William decided that that was
enough childbearing for her, even though he would have dearly

liked a son and heir. Cookworthy may not have travelled much at this time, but nevertheless, he was at home to travellers. These included a number of Naval Officers and a very different type of person, a potter by the name of André Duché from Savannah, Georgia. His parents were Huguenots who had escaped from France, in order to avoid the repercussions of the revocation of the Edict of Nantes. They had emigrated to Philadelphia, from which place André had subsequently moved to Georgia. He discovered china clay in the Indian Territory to the west of Virginia, recognising the material easily from Du Halde's description. Before visiting Cookworthy, Duché had run a number of experimental firing trials, and produced a quite reasonable porcelain. He brought Cookworthy samples both of the raw materials and the fired ware.

D'Entrecolles, when describing the raw materials used in the manufacture of porcelain, had called them by their Chinese names—petuntse—the material now known as china stone, and kaolin—the material now called china clay. When Cookworthy saw Duché's samples he was amazed—there in front of him were the true materials, both the kaolin and the petuntse. The appearance of the kaolin reminded him of something, and his mind winged back over the years until he remembered a certain bell-foundry and a certain material called pot growan. Duché left samples of both the clay and the stone with him, and went on to solicit custom for the clay and stone from potters who might be possibly interested. He left Cookworthy in a state of some excitement, fired with a determination that what Duché could find in America, he would try and find in Britain. A friend of his for many years had been the Quaker physician and surgeon, Dr. Richard Hingston, who at this time was in practice at Penryn, near Falmouth. It was to Dr. Hingston that Cookworthy wrote, describing Duché's visit, as follows:

I had lately with me (1744) the person who has discovered the China Earth. He had with him several samples of the china ware, which, I think, were equal to the Asiatic. It was found on the back of Virginia, where he was in quest of mines, and having read Du Halde, he discovered both the Petunse and the Caulin. He is gone for a cargo of it, having bought from the Indians the whole country where it rises.

They can import it for £13 per ton, and by that means afford their China as cheap as common stoneware; but they intend only to go about 30% under the Company.

From the fact that Duché came out of his way to visit Cookworthy, that gentleman's interest in the raw materials for porcelain must have become widely known. One of his sea-faring friends probably mentioned the matter in Georgia at the port of Savannah, on hearing that Duché had found clay and fired it successfully.

It may safely be said that Duché's visit marked a turning point in Cookworthy's life. He had seen the Oriental porcelain when he was in his 20's, he had read Du Halde in his 30's and seen the real materials in his 40's. From this time on, the great search began, over the length and breadth of Cornwall and parts of Devon. Cookworthy was sure that it was there waiting to be found. He remembered the bell-foundry, but he also remembered that John Astbury the Staffordshire potter had used a Cornish clay supplied him by a veterinary practitioner to improve the quality of his earthenware. This Cornish clay was in use in veterinary practice as far back as the late 1600's as a poulticing material. Cookworthy's mind was quick to equate the material used as a clay poultice with the material made into a clay paste in the bell-foundry, and then to equate both of these with the white material Duché had brought him.

It is often thought that Cookworthy had no experience whatsoever of ceramics prior to his development of a process for the manufacture of porcelain, but this is not absolutely true. Following the visit of Duché, Cookworthy entered into a business partnership in 1745 with Edward Heylin, formerly of the Bow Pottery, to set up a small works in Bristol manufacturing frit porcelain and glazes. It was their intention to obtain shipments of the china clay from Virginia, and to produce from this a better porcelain nearer to the true Oriental type. From what is known, the potting side was looked after by Heylin, whilst Cookworthy was more concerned with the business side, negotiating supplies of materials from various sources through his personal contacts. What finally became of this venture is not known, but it is known that Duché was unable to guarantee regular consignments of Virginian clay such as would be needed to keep a porcelain works going, due to several factors, including the breakdown of agreements with the Red Indians in whose territory the china clay was found and also to the weather delaying shipments of clay from the Atlantic seaboard ports. After 1746, Cookworthy was too busy with his own affairs to bother very much about the Bristol business and presumably it ground to a halt as a result of declining interest on the part of both the speculators.

III. THE GREAT QUEST

THE YEAR OF 1745 WAS ONE OF BOTH JOY AND SORROW for Cookworthy. By that year, he had done so well with the profits from the Notte Street Pharmacy, that he was able to buy out the Bevans' interests and become sole proprietor. In memory of the great help they had given him, however, he preserved the name of Bevan in the business, merely reversing the order to Cookworthy & Bevan, Dispensing Chemists. There were still Bevans who could have taken an interest in the business if they had so desired, these being the sons of the original founders of Plough Court, Timothy and Sylvanus Bevan, but one of these was a banker, being a founder of the banking firm of Barclay & Bevan, and the other, Joseph Gurney Bevan, was an author, and had no interest whatsoever in pharmacy. On his acquisition of the business, Cookworthy took his brother Philip in as a partner and his other brother Benjamin as a junior partner. Both brothers had served their time and become fully-fledged apothecaries in their own right by this time.

Early in June, Cookworthy paid a visit to Dr. Hingston at Penryn, and together, these friends rode westwards to see if they could discover the source of the clay. The noted antiquary and amateur mineralogist Dr. Borlase had just discovered a strange new mineral at Gew Graze, Kynance Cove on the Lizard, which he called the soapy rock. Borlase thought, in fact, that this soapy rock and the material known to the Chinese as kaolin were one and the same substance, but this was because he had not read his Du Halde properly, as Cookworthy had. D'Entrecolles had gone on, after describing the kaolin and petuntse, to describe another material which was also used by the Chinese to produce a type of porcelain. This type of porcelain, however, was inferior to that produced with kaolin and petuntse. Its principal ingredient was a material known to the Chinese as "hua hsih", literally "slippery stone". This, he said, was slippery or soapy to the touch, and Cookworthy was quick to recognise Dr. Borlase's soapy rock as being the same as "slippery stone". Nevertheless, both he and Dr. Hingston thought that a trip to the far west of Cornwall might not be unprofitable, and so they set out.

Their way from Penryn took them across the downs in the general direction of Helston, skirting on their way the tin mining district of Wendron. Wendron at this time was spattered with a number of small mines, together with a few larger ones. One of these latter, Trevenen Bal, they passed by on their way, and probably stopped to have a chat with the mine captain, Captain Tobias Martin, who was a devout Christian, interested, so it is believed, in religious reforms. The Bal at this time was very prosperous, and the two friends would have seen men wheeling the tinstone away from the skips, to where the bal maidens were waiting with their cobbing and spalling hammers to break the ore into small enough pieces to be put through the tin stamps. Even children were employed at this mine, and the sight of these little ones at work cannot have made the two friends very happy. Cookworthy's thoughts must have flown back to his little girls at home, and made him glad they would not have to labour at such a hard task.

As there were members of the Society of Friends at Helston, the two friends probably stopped to share a meal, a prayer, and a word of praise before going on with their journey. The roads were rough going for horses, and there was a limit to the number of miles one could be expected to cover in one day. From Helston, the two friends made for Godolphin. Here there was a friend of theirs, John Nancarrow, formerly of St. Agnes, a member of an old St. Agnes mining family who was now in charge of the Godolphin mines. In his charge were Godolphin Hill, West Godolphin, Great Work, and Wheal Grey. He was a man of some scientific knowledge, and a deep thinker. To reach Godolphin, the friends had to ride through more mining country, past the mines of Sithney and Carnmeal Downs. They would also have to pass what was the greatest of the Cornish mines at that time, Wheal Vor, which was already famous years before Dolcoath had begun to make a name for itself. When they reached Nancarrow's house, the three friends sat talking late into the night, until the fire's last embers had dwindled away into darkness and dust.

Cookworthy and Hingston stayed at Godolphin for several days, and whilst they were there, rode around the countryside looking for minerals. If they had but known it, the very material for which they were looking was there, right on Nancarrow's doorstep. Furthermore, Nancarrow himself knew that it was there, but did not know it was anything which would be likely to be of interest to them. When the three men sat down to break bread, they were more concerned about the spiritual state of the world than about clay and porcelain. At that time, there were many rumours of war and threats of disturbances, all of which were anathema to Quakers. It was the year of the Jacobite rising, known to the Scots as the "Glorious '45". Both Cookworthy and Hingston were pro-Hanoverian, disliking anything having any remote connections with Roman Catholicism, so that their sympathies were not with the Stuart Prince. Apart from the Jacobites, there was trouble in France and Spain and there were many possible threats to break the peace which was so dear to their hearts.

After leaving Godolphin, the two friends made their way through Crowan to Camborne, and thence to Redruth, St. Columb and Wadebridge to Camelford. From there, splitting up, Hingston returned to Penryn, whilst Cookworthy returned to Plymouth. Once again, as they made their way between Wadebridge and Camelford, they rode right past china clay without even realising that it was there. Clay was not finally discovered there, at the spot known as Stannon Marsh, until 1870, when several Quakers opened the first clay pit on the site of the present day well-known Stannon pit, which yields a useful potting clay. Cookworthy probably made his journey home skirting the bleak and desolate Bodmin Moor, by way of Launceston and Callington. Bodmin Moor was no place for a solitary horseman to be riding across, for, in those days, it was a haven for all manner of rogues, highwaymen, smugglers, tinkers and gipsies.

Poor Cookworthy! When he got home, it was to find his dear wife Sarah gravely ill, and all his physic and skill could not save her. It must have been agonising for him, as an apothecary, to have to sit there and be able to do nothing apart from relieving her of undue suffering. She died on July 11th, leaving behind her a grief stricken widower and five motherless girls, of whom the eldest was nine, whilst the others were seven, five and the twins just over two years old. Lydia, Sarah and Mary were old enough to have some realisation of their loss, but the twins were still too small to take in the full significance of what had happened. Cookworthy's unmarried sisters and his mother, then seventy-four, but still sprightly, had to take care of the children and try to make up for the love of their mother. It was fortunate for the children that their kin-folk were Quakers, devoted to sharing and caring. The very close-knit nature of Quaker life in those days ensured that in times of crisis and of need, all would pull together for the common cause.

For the next few months, Cookworthy hardly moved from home apart from going out to attend Quaker meetings. The loss of his wife was telling on him, and he was finally prevailed upon by his relatives and friends to go to stay for a month or two with his cousins and friends at Looe. Mrs. Cookworthy helped Philip run the business in his absence. It was late autumn by the time that he arrived there, but the weather was mild. After he had been there a while, his old spirits began to come back to him, and his mind began to dwell again on the quest for china clay. He began to take a few rides around the neighbourhood, keeping an eye open for any interesting minerals. He is said to have visited Duloe, St. Keyne, Dobwalls, Liskeard, St. Cleer and St. Neot. During his journeyings, for the third time he came within a short distance of china clay. On the moors between St. Neot and St. Cleer, china clay had been exposed in several places as a result of costcaning for tin, and had he only turned off from the main moorland paths he must surely have spotted it. The clay had already been used for ceramic purposes by a small pottery at Calstock during the 1730's, where it was used in a mixture with other clays to produce a whitish earthenware. The firing of the ware was never very successful, as there was too much specking, with deformation and fire cracking also occurring at times. By the time of Cookworthy's visit to the area, the pottery was either no longer functioning or was just about to cease operations.

In the following year, Cookworthy decided to take another trip to the far west of Cornwall in search of the elusive clay. He had asked in numerous places where pot growan could be found, and was always told "somewhere away to the west" or words to that effect. He had never met anyone who would actually acknowledge the existence of pot growan in their own district. Once again he made his way towards Helston and Godolphin, intending to use Nancarrow's house as a base for exploring the territory further west, such as the country around Marazion, Lands End and St. Just. If he had gone to Lands End, he might have discovered some china clay, as a little rather poorly coloured clay had been exposed as a result of mining operations at Balleswidden, Bartinney Downs and Tredinney Common, but this time fate was kinder to him, and he did not need to journey so far afield. It so happened that one of the mines under Nancarrow's supervision, Great Work, had taken delivery of a Newcomen steam engine, and this was now in operation, pumping water from the mine and winding to raise ore. Whilst staying with his friend, Nancarrow suggested to Cookworthy that he should pay a visit to the mine to see the methods of working, and also to see this Newcomen engine at work. Cookworthy was always interested in new inventions, and so he said that he would very much like to accompany his friend on a tour of inspection. Putting on protective smocks over their Quaker black, the two made a brief incursion into the upper levels of the mine workings. There, miners could be seen hard at work, stripped to the waist, hacking away with picks and chisels at the rock face, each of them streaked with perspiration and grimy from contact with the tinstone. Each miner had a tallow dip stuck on the front of his hard hat, by the dim light of which he could just about make out what he was doing. This scene underground, with the heat, lack of air and darkness, must have reminded Cookworthy of classical descriptions of the outer suburbs of Hell. No doubt he was glad to reach grass again and to breathe the fresh pure air of the hillside after the oppressive atmosphere below.

Having seen the ore being cut in the shallower levels, the two friends went on to see where it was being dressed. The operations at Great Work were similar to those at Trevenen Bal. A group of bal-maidens in their smock dresses covered with aprons were busy with heavy-looking cobbing hammers breaking the ore into manageable sized pieces. "'Tis no work for a woman, surely, this breaking of stones?" was Cookworthy's query, but his friend assured him that these Cornish women were as strong as any man,

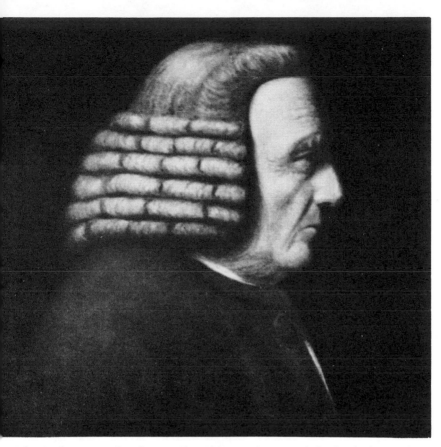

John Opie's portrait of William Cookworthy painted one year before his death in 1779

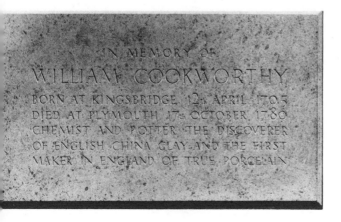

IN MEMORY OF

WILLIAM COOKWORTHY

BORN AT KINGSBRIDGE 12th APRIL 1705
DIED AT PLYMOUTH 17th OCTOBER 1780
CHEMIST AND POTTER THE DISCOVERER
OF ENGLISH CHINA CLAY AND THE FIRST
MAKER IN ENGLAND OF TRUE PORCELAIN

Tablet situated on south wall of St. Andrew's Church

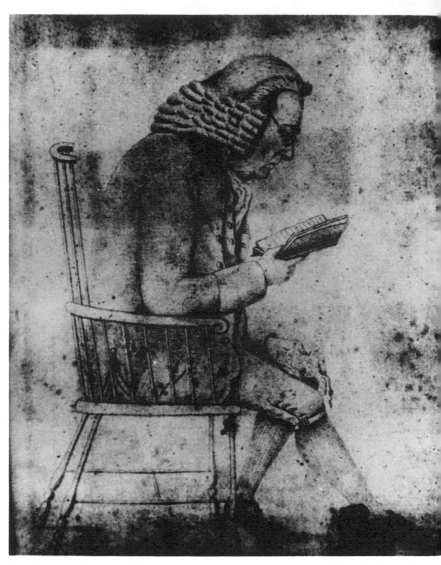

Opie's cartoon drawing of the ageing William Cookworthy, reading before the fire, when he was 74 years of age

and that each of them could break several tons of ore a day. Once again, Cookworthy was troubled to see children employed on the mine, though his friend set his mind at rest somewhat by telling him that they were only allowed to undertake the lighter tasks. Having seen all the other sights of the mine, the friends repaired to where the great engine was working away. It was here that Cookworthy's sharp eyes spotted some men making a white substance into a stiff paste to mend the furnaces and hearths of the engine. Surely this white substance looked familiar? His mind winged back over the years to the time of his visit to Fowey. With trembling hands, he pointed to the white material and asked Nancarrow, "Pray tell me, brother, what is the name of that white earth, and whence comes it?" Nancarrow, accustomed to seeing it in use without ever giving much thought to its nature and composition, was puzzled by his friend's sudden interest. "What, that? That is what they call the growan clay. 'Tis very useful for mending the furnaces of the fire engine [steam-engine] and for making bricks for the hearths. 'Tis to be had in great quantity not two miles from here. It costs nothing but the labour with which to dig it and bring it here."

On hearing this reply, Cookworthy fairly seethed with excitement. "My good friend, my dear, dear friend, I have searched for this very growan clay for ten years or more. Come, show me where it is to be had, and I will tell you what it is". They returned to Nancarrow's house so that Cookworthy could pick up his sample bag and auger, and then they climbed the 500' from the valley up to the working of Wheal Grey on the flanks of Tregonning Hill. With great eagerness, Cookworthy filled his bag with a sample of the clay, while his friend looked on in blank amazement, thinking that the heat of the mine must have affected his reasoning. Seeing the look on his friend's face, Cookworthy smiled, and said "No brother, I have not taken leave of my senses. This very earth, which you hold in such little esteem, is at this very moment being sought in every corner of Europe. 'Tis the caulin, just like that which Du Halde has written of. 'Tis the stuff of which real porcelain is made, the China Earth, as fine a sample of it as ever I saw. Now I must search for the petuntse, for caulin without petunse is like flesh without bones."

Still not completely recovered from his amazement, Nancarrow accompanied his friend while he examined each outcrop or area of exposed rock until at last he stopped, and began to take samples of a whitish rock. "'Tis the petunse of which I spoke before," explained Cookworthy. "Petun . . . Why, 'tis but the common moorstone, that everywhere abounds in these parts," said Nancarrow. On their way back down the hill Cookworthy explained in greater detail what had caused his initial excitement. Nancarrow still could hardly believe his ears, but he had a great enough regard for his friend's good sense not to dispute his word any further. Before returning home, Cookworthy made arrangements with the local landowner for the supply of trial quantities of the two materials, and got his friend Nancarrow to arrange for the loads to be carted to the nearest port of despatch, which was Porthleven. Having done this, Cookworthy made certain there was someone available with a boat at the little port who would be willing, at a fair price, to deliver the clay to Plymouth.

Once back home, he set about building a small kiln behind his premises in Notte Street, so as to be in readiness for when the first shipment of raw material was received. He was anxious to make a start with his experiments, but being methodical, he first sought to remind himself of Pere d'Entrecolles descriptions of the methods used in order to prepare the clay for use. Putting the clay matrix into a large mortar, he crushed it with a pestle until it had reached the consistency of a coarse powder. This he transferred into a large vat of water and stirred vigorously for some time with a spatula. He then let the suspension stand for a short while, in order to allow the coarser particles to settle. Then he poured the suspended clay off into another vat, taking care to leave all the sand and coarse sediment at the bottom of the first vat. Seeing some clay left mixed up with the sand, he added more water and restirred it, transferring a little more clay suspension into the second vat. The contents of this vat he allowed to stand undisturbed for several days until all the clay had settled at the bottom, and then he decanted all the clear water from the top. The resultant clayey paste he transferred into a series of moulds, which he put to dry in a warm place near the family cloam oven. He next turned his attention to the petuntse to prepare it, in turn, ready for the first trial batch. This proved to be a more difficult proposition. It was too hard to be conveniently ground down with a pestle and mortar, and remembering D'Entrecolles' description of the Chinese breaking it up with giant clubs or hammers, he followed the same procedure, breaking it first into smaller pieces and then crushing these until they were more or less a coarse granular powder. As a result of this experience, he decided that if he were ever to go into commercial production, he would have to acquire the use of a stone mill to grind it down, because of the length of time taken to do this by hand.

When the consignment arrived from Porthleven, he got the stone ground down properly and fired the first trial batch. On account of the high cost of coal delivered to Plymouth, he used wood to fire his kiln. The results were not a success in more ways than one. At first, he did not get his little kiln hot enough to fire the material properly, but after several attempts he got what he estimated to be more nearly the right temperature. The fired ware was not satisfactory, however. Not only this, but the smoke and fumes belching out of the chimney of his kiln right into Notte Street and Old Town Street did not prove popular with the general public, and so he decided to look around for a more suitable site for his firing trials. After some searching he located an old cloam kiln at Cockside [present day Coxside] which had been previously used by a small pottery producing brown earthenware. Being on slightly rising ground at the edge of Sutton Harbour, this was ideally situated in that the prevailing south westerly winds would blow the smoke and fumes away from the town. Furthermore, it was reasonably close to Cockside Wharf, so that consignments of clay or stone could be unloaded only a short distance away from it. He leased the cloam kiln and set about repairing and altering it as best he could. After this he gave instructions that when future consignments arrived at Plymouth from Porthleven, they should be forwarded on to Cockside Wharf.

The leasing of the Cockside cloam kiln marked the start of a new phase in Cookworthy's career. Hitherto, he had been first and foremost the apothecary. From this time, however, although he continued to exercise his normal profession with unabated diligence, much of his spare time was spent in trial firings at Cockside. He experimented with mixtures of china clay and china stone (petunse) in varying proportions—sometimes more stone than clay, sometimes more clay than stone. He produced ware of a type, but it did not really resemble porcelain, and was by no means good enough for commercial purposes. He was not to be put off by apparent failures, however; the more failures he had, the more determined he was that he would eventually triumph.

At this period, there were a number of cargoes landed at Plymouth which had been seized from foreign powers whilst on voyages from the Americas to Europe. Although these were sold legally on the open market, they were in reality goods obtained by legalised piracy, not having been paid for in the first place by the vendors. Some Quakers were involved in selling these goods, and there was at the time a conflict of consciences between them whether or not it was right for them to trade in goods obtained in such a manner. Cookworthy was against all traffic in the goods, and put his viewpoint to his friend Dr. Hingston in a letter, from which the following is an excerpt:

"We had lately very considerable sale here for the cargoes of the prizes taken by Admiral Martin's squadron, some time since, and also that from the "Elephant". J. Colesworthy was at this and bought a very large quantity of sugar on commission, as well as another Friend from London, whose name is Jonothan Gernal. We must not be at all surprised at this being, I am told, a settled matter that Friends may deal in prize goods, for on my attending F. Javel for being commercial in the purchase of the matter which he bought in partnership with Dr. Dicker and Lancelot Robinson, he pleaded, in his justification, that Friends at London were clearly of the opinion that there is no harm in it, and that John Hayward, a preacher, had given him the commission to buy prize and other stuffs. Brother F., who has done something in this way too, acquaints me that friend Wilson seems to be quite ignorant of anything wrong in the practice, and only advises in general that Friends should not work against their conviction. I am not interested or disposed to make any afflictions, and therefore shall only say that I hope that I shall be kept clear of it, as I believe it would bring a cloud over my mind."

Dear honest Cookworthy—he was a man who could have profited by buying cheap sugar for his pharmacy but he could not bring himself to purchase what he considered as stolen goods. He preferred to buy through the authorised channels, paying an honest price for goods honestly acquired. Few men of his time had such scruples about trading.

IV. FROM CHEMIST TO CERAMIST

WHILST HIS CERAMIC EXPERIMENTS CONTINUED TO BE unsuccessful, Cookworthy's pharmacy continued to be a success. As a result, Philip Cookworthy, now a partner in the business, decided that it was time for him to be married, and so it was that in 1747, at the age of 31, he married Rachel Morris. He was the first Cookworthy to marry into the Morris family. The stay-at-home Jacob, living all his life at Kingsbridge, was to marry Sarah Morris two years later in 1749, when he was 40 years old. 1747 was a year of mixed blessings for the Cookworthys. One of the saddest moments of the year was when baby Elizabeth, the twin sister to Susanna, contracted a serious infection which resulted in her death after only a short illness. The family were afraid that Susanna and the other children might have caught it, but if they did, they must have only contracted milder forms. Elizabeth was only four years old when she died. This was the second occasion when Cookworthy the apothecary had to look on in anguish, powerless to do anything to help. All the family missed 'Lizbeth, who had been a bright lively thing. Cookworthy himself, although he said little, was much saddened by her passing.

About this time, the Garrison (now called the Citadel) was requiring some repairs, and a consignment of stone was ordered from Cornwall. When the shipment arrived, Cookworthy was visiting the harbour on business, and spotted it being unloaded. Curiosity led him nearer, and he was amazed to find that it was china stone apparently similar to, if not better than that which he had obtained from Tregonning Hill. It seemed to contain less of the dark specks which were present in the Tregonning Hill stone, and which seemed to him to be the cause of specking in the fired ware. He asked one of the sailors on the quayside where the cargo hailed from, and was told Polmear. He was not exactly certain where this was, but further enquiries elicited the fact that it was near St. Austell. "That is nigh unto Fowey, then," said

Cookworthy. "Iss, 'tis so," replied the sailor. "Is the stone mined at Polmear?" Cookworthy enquired. "Naw, 'tis cut from up in the hills beyond," said the sailor. But beyond this he could tell Cookworthy nothing more. That worthy, however, was putting two and two together to make four. If china stone was always found near china clay, then where that stone came from, clay must be there also. He mentally resolved to go and make another search of the locality as soon as the occasion arose. He wrote of this to Dr. Hingston at Penryn, who replied that he would have another look for Cookworthy in the interim.

Early in 1748, Hingston was in the St. Austell area, and spotted what he thought was china clay on the Boconnoc family's estates, between St. Stephen and St. Austell. He reported this to his friend, who made arrangements shortly afterwards to investigate for himself. For some reason or other he did not go direct to St. Austell, but via Bodmin. Possibly he had a preaching engagement to fulfil on the way, or possibly he had a patient to visit at Lanhydrock House. In any case, going on from Bodmin he arrived at St. Columb Major. There he fell into conversation with a local gentleman, who offered to show him the parish church. When Cookworthy was taken up into the tower he noticed straight away that it was built of china stone. He therefore asked the gentleman whence it had been obtained, and was informed it was not an uncommon material locally, but that this particular batch of stone, as far as he could remember, had come from St. Stephen. As this was the place where Hingston had thought that he had found china clay, to St. Stephen Cookworthy went.

On his way there by way of Treviscoe, along a poorly defined moorland track, he saw a white scar on the hillside in the distance, but because there was no path branching off in that direction across the gorse and heather, he continued on towards the village. Having arrived at St. Stephen itself, he sought accommodation at the inn, as both he and his horse were very tired. The next morning, he got up early, and after breakfast went to look at the church. The china stone, being softer than granite and yet more durable than the killas, seemed to be in favour as a building material, and he wondered if he would find it used here, as well as at St. Columb. He asked permission to look round, and after viewing the interior was shown up into the tower. Yes—the tower, like that at St. Columb, *was* constructed of blocks of china stone! He looked at the general view of the countryside whilst he was there, as often the view from such an elevated building was better than could be obtained anywhere else in a village. To the north east, he saw once again the white scar in front of a round hillbrow. Turning to his companion, who had shown him over the church, he pointed to the scar and asked where it was. The man told him "'Tis King Pippin's Mount." Seeing Cookworthy's expression, he went on to explain "It do be properly called St. Stephens Beacon, but folk say that some old king be buried there in the burrow." "What about that white scar below the mount, then?" queried Cookworthy. "That—? 'Tis the mine—Tin Hill Mine they call it, though little tin they ever got from it. Some call it Carloggas." Cookworthy thanked his informant, and returning to the inn, paid his bill and called for his horse.

The track from the village towards the beacon was poorly defined, and at times Cookworthy thought that he had lost it, but he kept his horse's nose pointed in the general direction of the scar. As he came nearer, he found that the scar was where part of the hillside had been dug into, in an effort to locate a tin lode. Below the old workings in which the white clay was exposed was a small farmhouse, built of grey granite. Reining his horse in, Cookworthy dismounted, and tethering his mount to a bush, advanced across the moorland complete with his auger and sample bag. He found that the white was indeed clay, and whiter clay than that from Tregonning. Taking a good sample, he turned back down the hillside and knocked at the farmhouse door. A comfortably built middle aged woman came to the door. Doffing his tricorn hat, Cookworthy asked if the man of the house was at home. The woman said that if he would wait, she would fetch him. The farmer, when he appeared, turned out to be called Richard Yelland. At first he was a trifle suspicious of Cookworthy's intentions, but the latter's benevolent expression and gentle manner soon won him round and he became a loyal friend. Yelland explained that he was only a tenant farmer, and that to negotiate the mineral rights, Cookworthy would need to see Thomas Pitt of Boconnoc. This gentleman was the grandson of

"Diamond' Pitt", and nephew to William Pitt the Elder, "The Great Commoner" as he was known.

Whilst he was negotiating a proving lease of seven years on the Carloggas sett with Pitt, Cookworthy stayed at Carloggas Farm with the Yellands. Although only a humble farmhouse, the warm Cornish hospitality accorded to him, once he had built up the friendship, made up for the lack of other facilities. The Yellands were not Quakers, but they found Cookworthy's simple prayers quite acceptable to them. In the years that followed, Richard Yelland was to develop a considerable appreciation of the Quakers, through his contacts with Cookworthy. Being half Cornish himself, Cookworthy could understand the Cornish outlook on life better than the normal person from up country. Once Yelland knew exactly what it was that his visitor was looking for in the way of china clay and china stone, he proved very helpful with his knowledge of the locality. With his assistance, Cookworthy found that both the clay and the stone occurred in far greater quantities around St. Stephen than they did at Tregonning Hill. When he finally came to leave Carloggas, Cookworthy had engaged Richard Yelland to extract and process the clay and stone for him, and arrange for it to be shipped from Polmear direct to Cockside. The first two tiny pits opened by Yelland on Cookworthy's behalf were at Rescrowsa and Carloggas. In both cases a naturally occurring stream was available to be diverted in order to wash the clay. Whilst at Carloggas, Cookworthy had hit on the idea of using water to wash the clay before drying it, so as to save the cost of shipping a lot of unwanted quartz. This idea had come to him when he noticed that a stream running over clay was milky as the result of carrying away some of it. As he said, "Where Nature goes, man can follow." But to start with, he arranged for the first delivery to be unwashed, so that he could proceed with trials whilst Yelland was washing and drying a second batch.

On his return to Plymouth, he refined the St. Stephen clay and had the St. Stephen stone ground down. When fired, this looked much more like the porcelain than the Tregonning Clay had done, but there was still something wrong with it. He decided that as soon as he had the opportunity, he would visit some other potteries to see how they were going about the firing of their ware. He was hampered by the fact that no true hard porcelain was being manufactured in England at the time. He probably wished that he had paid more attention to the business which he called "the Bristol Affair"—his brief partnership with Heylin of the Bow Works at Bristol, as Heylin could have doubtlessly taught him a few tricks of the trade.

In 1750, Cookworthy's youngest brother Benjamin married Sarah Collins. He was then 32 years of age. Benjamin was destined to have one son, Joseph. After the death of Philip he was to become manager of the Notte Street Pharmacy, but this was all far away in the future. The pharmacy in 1750 continued to prosper, and more assistance was needed to cope with the work. Cookworthy at this stage of his career was putting in less time at the pharmacy and more at his kiln at Coxside. During 1750, he paid several visits to various ceramic works, including, so it is said, the Worcester Porcelain Works, which at this time was being run by two fellow Quakers, Dr. Thomas Wall and William Davies, who was an apothecary like Cookworthy; assisting them in their operations was a member of a well known potting family, Richard Holdship. The Worcester Tonquin Manufacture, as it was then known, was producing a kind of porcelain from glass frit and the Lizard soapstone. This was soft paste rather than hard. After Worcester, Cookworthy is said to have gone on to visit the Bow Works, where he had acquaintances.

It was about this time that Cookworthy made friends with two men destined to become famous—Captain James Cook, the explorer and Captain John Jervis of the *Foudroyant*, later to become Admiral Sir John Jervis. Both men put into Plymouth on occasions, and it was during their time ashore there that they met Cookworthy. They found him a very entertaining talker, with a considerable fund of knowledge on all sorts of subjects. Cookworthy was responsible for both men making sure that they had adequate stocks of fresh vegetables aboard, supplemented with sauerkraut, to combat that dreaded scourge of the Navy, scurvy. Cookworthy had a great many contacts at this time—largely due to the fact that once he had made a friend he kept him. Even some of the more autocratic Naval officers became his friends, and this in spite of the fact that he was a strict teetotaller and would never take spirits or wine with them. As one captain said, "One needs not wine to wag the tongue with Cookworthy." He was found useful when foreign visitors arrived at the port as he spoke several European languages fluently, and could always be relied on to act as a translator.

The period between 1750-1755 were quiet years in the life of William Cookworthy. During this time, he made a number of journeys around the countryside of both Cornwall and Devon. Around St. Stephen, he became a not unfamiliar figure, dressed in his black frock coat, bushy wig and tricorn hat, astride his grey mare. Apart from Richard Yelland, he had established a quite firm friendship with Thomas Pitt of Boconnoc, who was fascinated by what Cookworthy told him of his quest for clay and his attempts to find satisfactory means to fire it. At a later date, Pitt was to back Cookworthy financially in his Plymouth Porcelain Factory venture, but at this stage, everything was still experimental. Cookworthy's problem was not only to fire the ware, but also to glaze it successfully. He tried a large number of different types of glazes of the conventional sort, but their coefficient of expansion on firing was different to that of the body they were used to cover, and the result was poor finish to the glaze, cracking or crazing. As he confided to his friend Hingston:

"I am at a loss to know best how to set about the work of producing porcelain of a fit and proper nature. I have the caulin, which is the best that can be had, and I have the petunse, which I think is equal to the Chinese, and with these two I have both the flesh, the bones and the sinews, but to put flesh on bone to make a whole body, that is what perplexes me. There are times when I think that I shall, God willing, succeed in this enterprise, and other times when I wonder if 'tis destined for me to succeed. Such ware as I have made, when I attempt to apply to it a frit or glaze, seems to reject it, and at times the glaze will try to shrink more than the porcelain to which 'tis applied."

Whilst their father was going through all the various trials and tribulations that beset anyone making such experiments, the four surviving Cookworthy daughters were rapidly growing up. Lydia, Sarah and Mary were in their teens, whilst Susanna, the baby of the family was now quite a big girl. Both her father and her older sisters were very fond of Susanna, who was known to all the family as Sukey. Cookworthy, although he would have liked a son, was nevertheless very proud of his girls. "If I had a son, he would at sometime go away from me, but my dear girls will be a comfort to me in my later years. I must thank God that He has sought fit to leave me four blessings such as these." The four girls did, in fact, remain as a blessing to him in his later years. Even after they married, they still remained very close to him, and his sons-in-law came to feel far more like sons.

In 1755, Cookworthy renewed his lease of the Carloggas sett and took out a lease on another area on Trethosa moor. Richard Yelland still was looking after these clay producing interests for him. In the same year that the Carloggas lease was renewed, china clay was discovered in another part of Cornwall and had it not been for a quirk of fate, the discovery of this latter clay deposit might have been announced to the general public before Cookworthy made known his finds. This other deposit was the same one between St. Neot and St. Cleer which had been used by the defunct Calstock pottery, so that re-discovery would be a more accurate term. That year, a Mr. Horn from Staffordshire came to visit Dr. Borlase to see if he knew of any deposits of useful ceramic raw materials other than the Lizard soapstone deposits, which were then all under lease to various potters. Hearing of Horn's visit, a friend of Borlase's, John Trehawke of Liskeard, brought samples of the clay from the St. Neot deposit to show him, but Borlase, seeing that the material was nothing like Lizard soapstone in nature, rejected it as being of no interest. In this, he was short-sighted, as the soapstones have all been long worked out whilst the St. Neot deposit, now known as Park china clay pit, is still producing to this day.

Whilst Trehawke was rediscovering the St. Neot clay, Cookworthy was not idle in seeking out fresh sources for his own use. Crossing the old tracks across the moorlands at the southwestern edge of Dartmoor, he chanced to see clay exposed in the workings of the Bottle Hill mine and also a little further over at Hemerdon and Broomage. The clay, however, did not appear to be a very good colour, and the samples he took did not have a good fired colour either, so that he did not bother any more with them. Had he only travelled two miles further north and taken auger samples, he would have discovered there the much better quality deposits of

Lee Moor and Whitehall Yeo—which were destined, however, to sleep undisturbed for a further seventy-five years. It is interesting to speculate how long the Cornish clay deposits would have remained undiscovered if Cookworthy had found the Lee Moor clays before visiting Tregonning Hill. If he had found good clay so near to Plymouth, he certainly would not have been concerned to look so far afield as St. Stephen and Breage, and the whole history of the Cornish china clay industry might have been very different indeed.

In 1756, Cookworthy received a visitor of an unusual kind. Normally, apart from Quakers, he entertained Naval officers, merchantmen, other apothecaries, physicians and surgeons, but this man was none of these. He was what would be today called a civil engineer, and his name was John Smeaton. The two men, so different in many ways, one a quiet Devonian and the other a bustling Yorkshireman, became the firmest friends, and in fact Smeaton took up residence with the Cookworthys for three years. He had come to Devon to attempt to build a lighthouse on the infamous Eddystone Reef. Two previous structures had been built there, each of which were wrecked, and now there was no light there at all.

Smeaton commenced the work in 1756, using dove-tailed blocks of Portland stone for the tower instead of the ordinary square blocks and mortar. His idea was that if each block was keyed together, the whole would hold more firmly than any construction made of normal blocks. The two previous lighthouses had both been made of the latter and neither of them had stood up to the terrible weather experienced at times in the neighbourhood of the Eddystone reef. It was no easy task that he had undertaken—as the work could only be done in really calm weather, and this was the exception rather than the rule in such an exposed position. If Smeaton ever doubted that he would succeed, Cookworthy would reassure him with the words "If it is God's will, you will, and it must surely be God's will that no more men shall perish due to ships striking against that accursed reef". Cookworthy was a good judge of character, and he could see that the Yorkshireman had the necessary determination to carry the work through. His faith was justified when in 1759 the lighthouse was completed. The Cookworthys were sorry to lose the bluff

Yorkshireman, and he in turn was sorry to leave them. He did not lose touch with them altogether however, as he revisited them in 1775 whilst he was in Cornwall installing his modified 72″ Newcomen atmospheric engine at the Chacewater Mine in Gwennap, later known as Wheal Busy.

V. THE DAWN OF SUCCESS

IN 1758, COOKWORTHY AT LAST MANAGED A SUCCESSFUL firing of the Tregonning Hill clay and also had some quite reasonable results with the St. Stephen clay. Being a stickler for perfection, he was not yet fully satisfied with his work, but he was nevertheless pleased finally to have begun to make some progress, thanks to alterations he had made in the system of firing. As he confided to Dr. Hingston, "I thank God that at last I have succeeded in firing the china Earth that I got from Breag [Breage—or the Tregonning Hill area]. My problems with the glazing are being resolved. 'Tis best to make the glaze from the ground moorstone with some of the china earth, some lime and fern ash. This sits well in firing. and does not shrink or crack overmuch. Now I must set the china ware to some proper use, such as might be fit for what is required by the porcelain and china ware merchants. My porcelain must be both of use and of beauty."

In spite of this idea that any porcelain produced should be capable of being put to a useful purpose, he did in fact produce some purely ornamental pieces as well as coffee jugs, tea cups, teapots and the like. His early trial pieces between 1758-1760 were, however, largely of domestic porcelain, and unmarked. His use of the famous alchemists' sign for tin was not to come until later. This lack of marking has in the past led to some pieces of very early Cookworthy porcelain being viewed with suspicion, but most of the fraudulent "imitation Cookworthy" pieces are in fact marked with his sign. The best method for testing whether a piece is real Cookworthy or Champion hard paste, and not a soft paste imitation, is to subject it to ultra-violet light. The real article will then fluoresce to a deep purple, whilst the imitation piece will fluoresce a much lighter colour, which may be pink, lilac or lavender-mauve.

In 1759, his mother, Edith Cookworthy, died. She was by then a great age—88 or 89, having survived her husband for forty-one

49

years. She had seen her family rise from a state of extreme poverty after the death of her husband and the collapse of the South Sea Company to a state of moderate affluence. It gave her pleasure in her last years to know that three of her sons were working together in harmony in a common cause, and that each one was an eminently respected member of Quaker and Plymouth society. William, the eldest, never ceased to astonish her until the last. He had turned his hand to so many things and made a success of them that she viewed him with some awe, almost as if a hen had hatched out an ostrich. He had inherited much of his character from her, having her courage, tenacity and determination together with his father's sober and God fearing nature. This rather unusual combination doubtless made him the man he was.

For some time, Cookworthy had been driving himself rather hard. Philip had noticed this and attempted to restrain him. As Philip said: "My brother is his own hardest task master." It seemed as if he was almost engaged in a life or death struggle, such was his determination to finally draw his life's work to a successful conclusion. Even a man with a will as strong as Cookworthy's could only go on as long as his body would allow, however. Towards the end of 1759, he underwent a breakdown in health, and was forced at last, much against his grain, to consult a physician. Whether, in fact, he consulted Dr. Hingston is not known, but whoever it was that he saw recommended that he should go away somewhere quiet for a complete rest, preferably somewhere with sea air. At first, his brothers were afraid that Cookworthy would ignore this advice, but his own commonsense prevailed, and he set off early in 1760 to spend a quiet vacation with his cousins at Looe.

As before, after he had lost his wife, Dr. Looe did what was required, and the fresh sea air coupled with plenty of wholesome Cornish food began to restore the strength he had lost. When he had first arrived, Robert Debell confided to his wife "I fear that poor Will is in a sad decline," but in the ensuing weeks they began to see a marked change in him. At first, he was too tired to do much walking other than to attend the various Quaker meetings, but as his health picked up, he began to take quite a few walks, and the sparkle returned to his eyes. One of his regular walks was

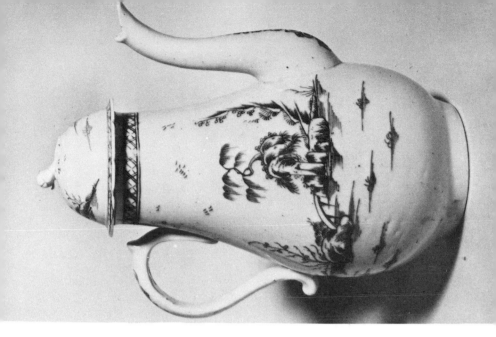

Coffee pot, made by
Cookworthy's factory at
Plymouth, decorated in underglaze
blue using Cornish cobalt.
Oriental design by one of Soqui's
pupils
Reproduced with the permission of
the City Art Gallery, Plymouth

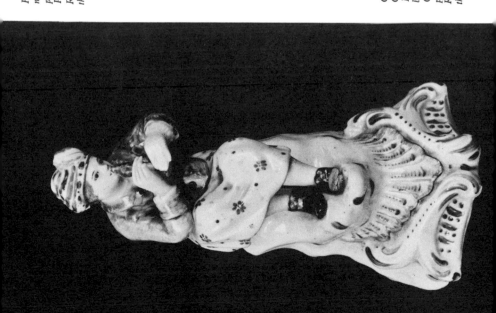

Figure of man playing a pipe,
modelled by Jacques Thibault and
produced by Cookworthy at the
Plymouth factory
Reproduced with the permission of
the City Art Gallery, Plymouth

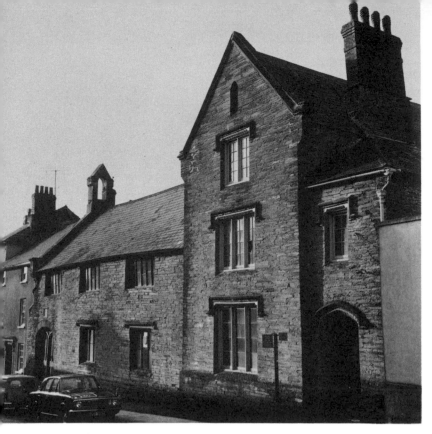

Kingsbridge school, where Cookworthy received some of his education, and which is now a Cookworthy museum
Photograph by J. A. Vaughan. Reproduced with the kind permission of English China Clays

View from Carloggas farm towards Cookworthy's clay pit at Rescrowsa

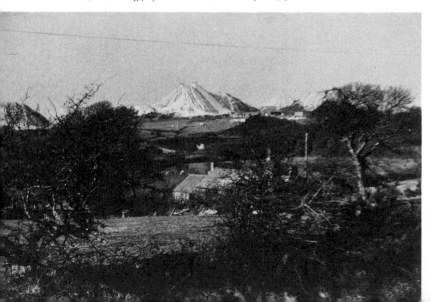

down to the harbour, where he would talk with the fishermen mending their nets or making lobster pots. He loved to watch the fishing boats putting out in the early morning and returning laden with fish just before nightfall. For him, it seemed like a link with those other fishermen who had toiled on the sea of Galilee, and had eventually become fishers of men.

At this time, Looe, in common with other ports on the south coast of the county, shipped barrels of salted pilchards and other fish to various Mediterranean ports, Cornish fish being greatly in demand amongst the Roman Catholics, who, because of religious obligations, were required to eat more fish than people in Protestant countries. Sailing barques and brigs would put out from Looe with cargoes for Genoa, Naples and other ports. Watching them load the barrels of fish and then load kegs of fresh water for the voyage, Cookworthy fell to meditating on the unprofitability of carrying water on board, occupying space which could have taken cargoes, when all around the ships there was an ocean full of water, even if salt. He knew from what Philip and other seafarers had told him that the water, which started out fresh at the beginning of the voyage might be anything but fresh before the ship arrived in another port where supplies could be replenished. He knew also, that foul water caused various stomach upsets and other internal disorders, although, in common with most other scientific gentlemen of his time, he was not aware of the true cause for such disorders. The existence of microbes and bacteria was quite unknown at that time, illnesses being thought to be caused by what were known as "humours". It was the foul humours in polluted drinking water which sometimes led to epidemics of cholera or plague, and it was the foul humours given off from marshes and swamps that gave rise to the swamp fever suffered by the early colonial settlers in the Southern States of America.

Salt water to fresh water, an ideal solution to the drinking water problem, but how? It could be done on shore in a laboratory, but on board ship was a different matter. Cookworthy gave the matter deep thought, and then went to discuss with ships' masters and other seafarers the feasibility or otherwise of his ideas. Gradually a method crystallised itself in his mind, and asking for pen and paper, he set it down. He realised how useful his invention

could be to naval vessels engaged in active service without hope
of putting regularly into port to replenish water supplies. He also
saw how useful it might prove to the East Indiamen, such as
Philip had sailed on. He resolved, on his return to Plymouth, to
offer his invention to both the Navy and the merchant service.*

Cookworthy returned to Plymouth with renewed vigour,
prepared to make a fresh start of firing trials at his kiln at Cockside. 1760 was to prove a happier year for him, after all, after the
inauspicious start it had made. During the year, he learned that
the Longton Hall Pottery in Staffordshire was closing down, and
that various items of equipment were up for sale. He made the
journey there and bought the figure moulds, previously used for
producing soft paste porcelain figurines, together with other
moulds and equipment suitable for use in a porcelain manufactory. He then engaged the services of the French moulder and
designer, Jacques Thibault. This turbulent character, whose name
is sometimes spelt Tebo phonetically, had previously worked
with Cookworthy's Quaker acquaintances, Dr. Wall and W.
Davies at the Worcester Tonquin Manufactory, and had also
worked at Bow. Both of these establishments found him to be
very temperamental and difficult, if not impossible, to handle,
and yet he worked in perfect harmony with Cookworthy for
twelve years. This was largely due to Cookworthy's ability to
make friends and keep friends with all sorts and conditions of
men. Thibault went on to work for Wedgwood in 1774 after
Cookworthy relinquished his interest in porcelain manufacture,
but this association was of very short duration, Wedgwood
declaring to a friend of his "that damned Frenchman is impossible".

In the same year that Thibault came to work for Cookworthy,
his second eldest daughter, Sarah, then 22 years of age, married
Francis Fox, He was one of the sons of the well known Quaker
George Fox of Biscovey, near Par, in Cornwall. Francis's mother
was related to Edith Cookworthy, being Anna Debell of Looe
prior to her marriage. Sarah's marriage was not destined to be of
long duration, but she bore her husband three children, Sarah,

---

* His hand-written method for producing distilled water from salt water on board ship
is still preserved at the Plymouth City Museum.

William and Francis before his untimely death. Francis Fox the younger was later to run the Notte Street Pharmacy until his death in 1812.

Once having acquired both the moulds and the modeller, Cookworthy began to produce his first figurines, obviously having forgotten what he had once said about porcelain being both of use and of beauty. He was keen to see what sort of figurines he could produce in hard paste, the Longton Hall ones having been made only in soft paste. The moulds acquired from Longton included a set of "The Continents"; a set of rustic figures, including a bagpiper, a shepherdess, a goatherd and a milkmaid; a set of "The Seasons"; a set of infant "Seasons"; a "Boy with Dolphin"; cherubs garlanding a goat and some classical animals such as sphinxes, lions, lionesses, and a mother ewe with lamb. When Thibault produced figurines from these moulds for Cookworthy, he impressed on their bases the mark T°. A great number were produced using the Longton moulds, some in plain white, after the manner of the classical "blanc de Chine", whilst others were decorated with enamel colours. The white pieces show that they were produced quite early in the Cookworthy-Thibault association, as there are various defects in them, such as sagging, fire cracks, foxing or specking due to the presence of biotite or ferruginous minerals in the clay used for the body.

In 1762, Mary, the third of the Cookworthy girls married a Quaker physician, Dr. Benjamin Hobson. She was then 22, whilst he was about thirty. Like her sister Sarah, she was not to enjoy married life for very long, as her "poor sweet Ben" died only three or four years after her marriage. She had one daughter by him, but this child died in infancy. The loss of Ben Hobson was a tragedy not only to Mary but to the other Cookworthys as well, as during the short period in which he had been associated with the family, they had all learned to love him. His father-in-law said of him with great tenderness, on his passing "He saved others, himself he could not save".

In 1763, Cookworthy's translation out of Latin of Emmanuel Swedenborg's *Doctrine of Life* was published. This was produced as a result of his contact with Swedenborg, who was then resident in London. How Cookworthy found time, amidst all his other activities, to make friends with such a man and then translate such a weighty work, remains an unsolved mystery, but of course he was a man who was well nigh indefatigable in the pursuit of knowledge, and who, from the time of his apprenticeship with the Bevans was accustomed to burning the candle at both ends— and in the middle as well, if occasion demanded. In later years, Cookworthy was to become an able exponent of the Sweden- borgian philosophy. One of those to whom he expounded his ideas was a certain James Woods, a brewer, who, however, seemed to be left with somewhat mixed feelings afterwards. Captain Jervis, however, proved to be a more intelligent listener. After having the Doctrine of Life explained to him, he returned to his ship, the *Foudroyant*, in such a state of mental excitement that he felt that he must get his chaplain, the Revd. M. Gardner, out of bed to tell him of it. This gentleman took unkindly to the Captain's disturbing his sleep, and proceeded to give an anti- Swedenborgian sermon, upon hearing which Jervis said "Hold your tongue, sir. If I delight in hearing Mr. Cookworthy's instruction, I did not come here to receive a sermon from you, I came only to make you participate in my pleasure".

The period 1763-64 saw Cookworthy busy with his Cornish china clay and china stone. This, together with pharmaceutical research, Swedenborgian studies and his duties as a Quaker minister, not to mention regular visits from his various seafaring friends, must have kept him very busy indeed. The Looe air, how- ever, must have been a very potent tonic, because his energy seemed to be almost boundless. He was keeping Thibault busy at Cockside with experimental firings, whilst still not neglecting any of his other interests.

Whilst Cookworthy was busy with his supplies of Cornish clay, his friend and fellow Quaker, the young Richard Champion, received a sample of another clay called "unacre", obtained from the Cherokee Indian country of South Carolina. Champion was a man of many and varied interests, instituting improvements in berthing facilities at Bristol Docks for example at the age of twenty. A year later he inherited a shipping business dealing directly with Charleston in South Carolina. Although he was interested in all things artistic he did not turn his attention to the manufacture of porcelain until he received samples of American clay, whereupon he took over a disused pottery at Castle Hill. Thomas Frank, formerly at Worcester, was appointed as his foreman. He did not achieve great success with the Cherokee clay, because he did not have any china stone to go with it, but he did succeed in making a sort of semi-porcelain, with glass frit as the other ingredient.

In 1765, Cookworthy visited both Bristol and Worcester. He took with him to Bristol samples of St. Stephen china clay and china stone. These two materials were still giving him trouble, although he had succeeded in producing some figurines with them. When he confided his problems to Champion, that young man must have discussed them with his foreman, an old hand at making soft paste porcelain. That worthy suggested Cookworthy's kiln might be at fault, and pointed out that there was an old disused glasshouse kiln which would probably be better. Cookworthy took a short lease of the kiln and tried firing his clay and stone in it. He was quite elated with the successful results. Taking a good note of the design of the Bristol glass kiln, he hurried back to Plymouth and began building a new kiln to the same design at his Cockside pottery.

At this juncture, Cookworthy stopped and took a long cool look at what he had achieved. One thing concerned him, and that was whether he would live long enough to see his process through to a full manufacture. Up to this time, he had written little concerning his researches, although he had written something of his spiritual experiences as a Quaker. In many ways, he regarded his spiritual life as being of greater importance than what he referred to as "the china affair". Even when he was fully involved with his experiments, his Quaker activities came first. Now, however, he suddenly felt a pressing need to preserve his invention in writing, in case His Lord should claim him before he was ready. To this end, he wrote down an account of his experiences, and the following is an extract from this account.

"It is now nearly twenty years since I discovered that the ingredients used by the Chinese in the composition of their porcelain were to be got, in immense quantities in the County of Cornwall, and as I have, since that time, by abundance of experiments clearly proved this to the entire satisfaction of many ingenious men, I was willing that this discovery might be preserved to posterity, if I should not live to carry it to a manufacture. The petunse gives the ware transparency and mellowness, and is used for glazing it. The stone of the petunse is a species of granite or as we in the west call it, "moorstone". I first discovered it in the parish of Germo, in a hill called Tregonnin Hill. That whole country in depth is of this stone. It reaches east and west from Breag to Germo, and north to south from Tregonnin Hill to the sea. From the cliffs, some of this stone hath been brought to Plymouth, where it was used in the casemates of the Garrison; but I think the best quarries are in Tregonnin Hill. The stone is compounded of small pellucid gravel and a whitish matter, which indeed is caulin petrified, and as the caulin of the Tregonnin Hill hath abundance of micae in it, this stone hath them also. If the stone is taken a fathom or two from the surface, where the rock is quite solid, it is stained with an abundance of green spots, which are very apparent when it is melted. This is the circumstance noticed by the Jesuits, who observe that the stones which have most of this quality are the most proper for the preparation of glaze. A vein of this kind in Tregonnin Hill is so much so that it makes an excellent glaze without the addition of vitrescent ingredients. The caulin is a white talcy earth, found in our granite country in both the counties of Devon and Cornwall. It lies in different depths below the surface beneath a cover of burden. It is by no means a regular stratum, but is rather in bunches, or heaps. There are inexhaustible stores of this caulin in the two western counties. The use it's commonly put to is in mending the furnaces and the fireplaces of the fire engines (i.e. steam pumping engines) for which 'tis very proper. The sort I have chiefly tried is what is got from the side of Tregonnin Hill, where there are several pits of it. The caulin is prepared for manufacture by pouring a large quantity of water so that it may not, when dissolved, be of so thick a consistence as to suspend the micae. Let it settle about ten minutes, and pour off the water and dry it. The water with which 'tis to be washed ought to be pure, without any metallic or calcareous mixture. I have later discovered that in the neighbourhood of the parish of St. Stephens, in

Cornwall, there are immense quantities of both the petunse stone and the caulin, and which, I believe, may be more commodiously and advantageously wrought than those from the Tregonnin Hill, as by the experiments I have made on them, they produce a much whiter body and do not shrink so much by far in baking, nor take stains so readily from the fire. The parish of Dennis, the next to St. Stephens, I believe, has both the ingredients in plenty in it. I know of two quarries of the stone, one is just above St. Stephens, the other is called Caluggas (Carloggas) somewhat more than a mile from it, and appears to be the finer stone."

Having unburdened himself in this manner, Cookworthy settled down to the task of patenting his process. If it was not patented, it would soon be pirated by the major Staffordshire potters who would, in their own parlance, "take all and give nought". Cookworthy was not interested in personal financial gain, but was interested in leaving his daughters well provided for, so that he was bound to endeavour to obtain a degree of commercial success from his discoveries. He was not, like Wedgwood and Spode, first and foremost a man of business. He was first a Quaker, then a chemist, then a potter and only lastly a business man. It says something for the courage of the man that he was prepared, through his patent and its consequences, to stand up to such men as Josiah Wedgwood I. This gentleman would dearly have liked supplies of china clay not for the manufacturing of porcelain, but for the improvement of his earthenware, and in particular his Queen's Ware and the celebrated Jasper. Wedgwood had seen samples of the Cherokee clay, a year or so before, and had sent an agent out to South Carolina to procure a consignment for him. This the agent did, and the Cherokee clay was used for the next batches of jasper. Wedgwood himself was in two minds as to whether he should advertise the fact that the Cherokee clay, which was in very limited supply, had been used for the jasper, but his problem was that he could not be certain of getting further supplies, failing which he would have to revert to his old formula for this type of ware. China clay obtained from Red Indian country was a rather uncertain commodity, as Cookworthy and Heylin had found before him.

During the next two years, Cookworthy did not travel very far afield, apart from a visit to make certain all was well with production at his china pits at St. Stephen. He had much to do, and little time to do it in. Apart from preparing his patent, he had to make plans for the establishment of a factory in which to produce his porcelain. To do this, he had to be sure that he would have enough capital to finance the operation. Although he was reasonably prosperous, he did not have the total amount of money in reserve which might be needed, so he had to secure financial backing. He approached several of his friends and relations, and received promises of financial assistance from Thomas Pitt of Boconnoc, from his brother-in-law, Thomas Were, a Woollen manufacturer of Wellington in Somerset, and from Richard Champion.

The kilns at Cockside were satisfactory, since their modification for the firing of the porcelain, but there was insufficient room there for large scale moulding, modelling and decoration of ware. New premises needed to be found so that he could accommodate the required staff, and these premises needed to be near the kilns, so that the whole manufacturing complex could be confined to a given area, with the clay arriving at Cockside wharf, being delivered to the Cockside Kilnhouse and the fired ware being finished at the factory. Finally, he secured premises at the rear of Weeke's House, in Higher Vintry Ward which could accommodate some fifty or more persons engaged in their work. His life's ambitions looked like being achieved. The only note of sadness to mar the family's happiness was when Francis Fox died in 1766, at the age of 30, leaving his wife Sarah to cope with three small children. Francis had been a good father and a good son-in-law, and his passing left a blank space in the family impossible to fill. Early death was by no means uncommon in those days however, and the Cookworthys had had their share of it. As Cookworthy said, however "when the harvest is ripe and ready, no-one can deflect the scythe of the reaper".

The Cookworthy girls were lucky in their choice of husbands, all marrying very good, kind men, but unlucky in that two of them were to be early widows. The only one of the three daughters to marry who did enjoy a full married life was Sukey (Susanna) Her husband, George Harrison, whom she did not marry until

she was 33 years old, outlived her by seventeen years, finally
dying at the ripe old age of eighty.

VI. FULFILMENT

URING 1767, COOKWORTHY PUT THE FINISHING TOUCHES to his patent, and got everything ready for the official opening of his porcelain factory. He set about engaging staff, the nucleus of which were drawn from the Bow Porcelain factory. Whether Edward Heylin, formerly of Bow and partner with Cookworthy in his ill-fated 1745 frit porcelain venture at Bristol, was associated with the new enterprise, is not known, but with his previous experience he would have been an obvious choice. John Brittan, who had been engaged in this Bristol venture in 1750, was foreman at Plymouth. Cookworthy already had the services of Thibault, the modeller and assembler, but he also needed ceramic artists to decorate the ware. He had done a little early blue decoration himself, using Cornish cobalt under the glaze, but this was all of a rather primitive nature—a few sprigs of flowers and leaves or simple floral-based designs, and would not have been acceptable as competition to the elaborately designed and decorated French, Italian, German and Chinese porcelains. He therefore secured the services of another Frenchman, Henri Saqui, formerly employed at the Sevres porcelain factory. His penchant was the modelling and painting of exotic birds of no known and recognizable ornithological species, but which appeared to be a blend of pheasant, peacock and bird of paradise*. Even at the beginning, there was work for more than one decorator, and so Cookworthy engaged some apprentices— two Cornish boys, Henry Bone and William Stephens, together with a young man from Plymouth, Philip James. Henry Bone was only thirteen when he joined the factory. Born in Truro in 1755, he moved to Plymouth with his parents in 1765 and was later to become famous as a miniature painter and painter in enamels to George IV.

*The two famous coloured "pheasants" are examples of his workmanship, both now housed in the Plymouth City Museum.

Cookworthy's patent was issued on March 17th 1768 [No. 898] and the following is an abridged version:

MANUFACTURE OF PORCELAIN

"To all people to whom these presents shall come, I William Cookworthy, of Plymouth, in the County of Devon, chemist, send greeting. Whereas his most gracious Majesty King George the Third, by letters patent bearing date at Westminster, the seventeenth day of March now last past, did give and grant unto me, the said William Cookworthy, my executors, administrators and assignees, that I, the said William Cookworthy etc. should make, use, exercise and vend a kind of porcelain, newly invented by me, composed of moor stone or growan and growan clay, within that part of His Majesty's Kingdom of Great Britain, called England, his Domain of Wales and town of Berwick-upon-Tweed, and that I should lawfully have and enjoy the whole profit, benefit, commodity and advantage from time to time accruing and arising by reason of the said invention until the full end and term of fourteen years from the date of the said letters patent.

"Now know ye that I, the said William Cookworthy, do by this my deed in writing, declare the nature of my said invention and the quality of the materials and the manner in which the same is performed, which is as followeth:-

"The materials of which the body of the said porcelain is composed are a stone and earth or clay. The stone is known in the counties of Devon & Cornwall by the names of moorstone and growan, which stones are generally composed of grains of stone or gravel of a white or whitish colour, with a mixture of talcy shining particles. This gravel and these particles are cemented together by a petrified clay into very solid rocks, and immense quantities of them are found in both the above mentioned counties. All these stones, exposed to a violent fire, melt without the addition of fluxes into a semi-transparent glass, differing in clearness and beauty according to the purity of the stone. The earth or clay, for the most part, lies in the valleys where the stone forms the hills. This earth is frequently very white, though sometimes of a yellowish or cream colour. It generally arises with a large mixture of talcy mica or spangles and a semi-transparent whitish gravel. Some sorts have little or none of the mica or spangles, but the best clay for making porcelain always abounds in mica or spangles. The stone is prepared by levigation, in a potter's mill in water, in the usual way, to a very fine powder. The clay is prepared by diluting it with water until the mixture is rendered sufficiently thin for the gravel and mica to subside, the white water containing the clay is then poured or left to run off from the subsided mica and gravel into proper vessels or reservoirs, and after it has settled for a day or two, the clear water above it is to be then poured or drawn off, and the clay or earth reduced to a proper consistence by the common methods of exposing it to the sun and air, or laying it on chalk. This earth or clay gives the ware its whiteness and infusibility as the stone doth its transparence and mellowness; they are therefore to be mixed in different proportions as the ware is intended to be a more or less transparent, and the mixture is to be performed in the method used by potters and well known (viz. by diluting the materials in water, passing the mixture through a fine sieve and reducing it to a paste of a proper consistence for working, in the way directed for the preparation of the clay). This paste is to be formed into vessels, and these vessels when biscuited are to be dipped in the glaze, which is prepared of the levigated stone with the addition of lime and fern ashes, or an earth called magnesia alba, in such quantities as may make it properly fusible and transparent when it has received a due degree of fire in the second baking.

WILLIAM L. S. COOKWORTHY

Signed, sealed and delivered by the said William Cookworthy in the presence of

George Leach   J. Stove

When the factory finally opened, it employed between fifty and sixty persons in all. Output fell into two categories, useful domestic porcelain and more artistic decorative porcelain pieces. Although the figurines produced are very lovely, to appreciate fully the quality of the porcelain and also its defects, it is necessary to look at the more simple blue on white or plain white pieces. These were freer of the firing defects noticeable in the very early experimental Cookworthy pieces—spiral wreathing, caused by the thrower's hand as he guided the pot on the wheel, faults in firing such as cracks, or fissures in the paste, deformation, misshapen pieces, iron specking or foxing, peppering (due to being overfired) and smoke staining. The best examples of the 1768-1772 white Cookworthy possess a smooth finish and good blue-white colour with clear rather than blurred under-glaze decoration. Cookworthy's under-glaze blue always tended to be rather darker than the Nankin blue he was trying to reproduce. In the earliest pieces the blue was very dark, almost indigo to black, but in the later pieces a slightly less dark blue was obtained something like a dark ultramarine or navy blue.

The "useful pieces" included a number of cider mugs, some of which were bell-shaped and others straight sided. There were also sauceboats, sweetmeat dishes, cream dishes, coffee pots, teapots, cream jugs, and very rarely, cups and saucers. Cookworthy experienced difficulties in producing saucers which we should recognise as such—being more like very shallow dishes. As far as is known, he never succeeded in mastering the technique of producing porcelain plates. The pieces were decorated in a great variety of styles, and were obviously executed by several different artists, as the techniques employed show. The most common type of decorations were the pseudo-Chinese type, with pagodas, willow trees, various exotic, imaginary flowers and Oriental landscapes, but there were also some pieces produced with decorations in the "French" manner—delicate floral wreaths, interlacing greenery and classical landscapes, usually with ruins in the background. Some of these were also decorated with the type of exotic bird characteristic of Henri Saqui, and it is assumed that these pieces were therefore decorated by him. Apart from the pseudo-Chinese and the French types of decorations, there were also some pieces produced with characteristic formal floral patterns showing various types of daises, marguerites, calendulas, roses, forget-me-nots and occasionally violets.

The ornamental pieces consist of figurines, animal pieces, urns and vases. Although the Longton Hall moulds, bought in 1760, were used to produce the majority of the figures, there were quite a few pieces copied from the production of other works such as Bow, Chelsea and Worcester. With a number of former Bow employees at the factory, it was not surprising to find copying of pieces from there. Notable amongst these were some statuettes, including those of the celebrated actor Woodward and Kitty Clive. These were produced first at Bow around 1758 and then reproduced at Plymouth about 1770. The pieces which were not copies of other works' productions included a number of animal and bird pieces—lions, lionesses, heifers, lambs, sheep, dogs, sphinxes, hares, finches and above all the exotic birds of Henri Saqui. Some of the pieces were modelled by Thibault and decorated by Saqui, but there were other modellers at work also— as Thibault had apprentices working under him. Some modelling was apparently done outside the factory, as there was a record of a Mrs. James who specialised in the modelling of animals. The pug is said to be her work. One animal noticeably absent was the domestic cat. There were big cats in the form of lions, but no ordinary cats, and yet the cat was an ordinary domestic pet. One wonders whether Mrs. James was an ailurophobe. Cookworthy apparently was not, as a late drawing showed him with a cat at his feet. The reason was more likely that cats were considered to be too ordinary to be worth modelling. In the same way, there were few models of dogs, apart from the pug.

Trade was brisk for the products of the factory—it being the only one making true hard paste. Pieces went abroad, quite a few going to North America, and at one period these were being produced faster than the decorators could cope with them. As a result of this, Cookworthy asked Champion to advertise for decorators for him in the hopes of enticing a few workers to move to Plymouth from Worcester. The advertisement was published in the *Worcester Journal* of February 22nd 1770, and ran as follows:

"China painters wanted for the Plymouth new invented patent porcelain manufactory. A number of sober, ingenious artists capable of painting in enamel or blue may hear of constant employment by sending their proposals to Thomas Frank in Castle Street, Bristol.

In the same year, 1770, Cookworthy signed a new lease of 99 years on the Carloggas setts, and obviously did not intend ceasing porcelain production immediately. Some authorities say that the factory closed in 1770, others in 1772, but the latter date appears to be the correct one as production was still coming from the factory up to that date. The boom year of 1770, however, did not follow on into 1771, by which time demand was falling off. What really brought about the closure of the factory was economic considerations, as Cookworthy's financial resources were not unlimited. There were originally fourteen shares issued for the factory; of these only three were held by Cookworthy himself, the remainder being divided between Thomas Pitt, Richard Champion and Thomas Were (Cookworthy's brother-in-law). If all the articles produced had been saleable, the factory might have continued longer than it did. There were a great number of costly rejects, however. On some pieces the ratio of rejects was one out of three, although others were more trouble free. The pieces which were most expensive to produce in terms of the hours involved in modelling, firing and decorating, were the ones most prone to rejection, for figures sagged or warped in firing or had too many firecracks in them to be saleable. Towards the end of 1771, the fires in the kilns were allowed to go out for the last time, although some work continued after this, decorating pieces already made. Those workers willing to make the move were transferred to Champion's factory at Bristol, a few at a time, until the day arrived when the erstwhile bustling manufactory was silent and deserted. All the key workers transferred to Bristol—Jacques Thibault, Henri Saqui, Henry Bone and William Stephens.

Not all the pieces produced at Plymouth were marked alike, and some were not marked at all—these being early pieces. The most characteristic mark was the alchemist's symbol for tin, applied under the glaze in blue, or enamelled on afterwards over the glaze in rose pink or reddish brown. A few pieces bore the coat of arms of Plymouth, and amongst the other marks were the T° (denoting a piece modelled by Jacques Thibault), W.C., & C.F. (Cookworthy Fecit). Not so much a mark as an inscription is found on some pieces made at a time when the move to Bristol was imminent—these being inscribed "Mr. Wm. Cookworthy's Factory, Plymouth". Cookworthy pieces manufactured at Bristol bore a plain + with or without a number indicating the decorator, a B for Bristol, or in the later pieces produced by Champion crossed swords in an imitation of the Meissen mark.

One would have thought that what with the porcelain factory, the pharmacy and his Quaker ministry, Cookworthy would not have been able to find time to entertain during this period, but such was not the case. His house was still open to all manner of Naval officers and men, merchantmen and the like, no matter how busy he was. His saying was "One should always have time for one's friends. If one has not, then there is something amiss with one's soul." An example of this great hospitality occurred in 1768 at the time when the porcelain factory was just opening, and Cookworthy was exceedingly busy. At this time, the factory was producing more fired ware and figurines than there were decorators available. The visitors who were, nevertheless, made welcome in the Cookworthy household, were his old friend Captain James Cook, together with Sir Joseph Banks and Dr. Daniel Solander. They were due to leave Plymouth on board the *Endeavour* in order to observe the transit of Venus at Otaheite in 1769. Cookworthy was interested in astronomy, as he was in all other forms of natural science, and would dearly have liked to have gone with them, but his duty lay with his flock, and so he contented himself with holding learned discussions with the great navigator, the scientist and the astronomer before they sailed.

Cookworthy was not to see his friend for several years. After leaving Plymouth on their voyage to Otaheite, the explorers took a course taking in Cape Horn, the Society Islands, New Zealand, Eastern Australia, Papua, the East Indies and the Cape of Good Hope before arriving back at Plymouth. In 1772, just as the porcelain factory was closing down, Cookworthy saw his friend again, this time on the eve of Cook's second voyage of discovery, which was to take him via West Africa and the Cape of Good Hope down to the fringes of Antarctica before turning in the direction of New Zealand. He then dipped down towards Antarctica again before coming up to the Society Islands. He explored the straits between the North and South Islands of New Zealand and proved them navigable, and then returned via Cape Horn, South Georgia and South Africa. Cookworthy saw him on his return, and was overjoyed to hear of all he had seen and discovered.

VII. BRISTOL FASHION

IT HAS NEVER BEEN FULLY UNDERSTOOD WHY COOKWORTHY transferred his manufacture of porcelain to Bristol. Plymouth was so much nearer the source of the basic raw materials of china clay and china stone, that one would have thought that if Cookworthy had wanted to relinquish responsibility for the works, it would have been better for Champion to have moved his works to Plymouth. His Bristol pottery had not been an outstanding success hitherto, as he had been unable to obtain all the American china clay he wanted, and had found difficulties at first in using the Cornish materials supplied to him by Cookworthy. It has been said that Cookworthy was feeling his advancing years by this time—he was 67, and had led a very active life, covering more ground than most of his contemporaries amongst the Society of Friends. He wished to devote more time to his family and his Quaker ministry, which he could not have done whilst still being responsible for the operation of the factory.

As has been stated, the move to Bristol was accomplished piecemeal, the first nucleus arriving at Castle Green in 1771, including the principal modellers and decorators. The bulk of the Longton Hall moulds were transferred at this time, the remainder going to Bristol with the last of the Plymouth staff. By the end of 1772, all the old Plymouth hands who had been willing to move had been installed at the new factory. Both the Frenchmen moved to Bristol initially, but neither Thibault or Saqui would stay on to work with Champion after Cookworthy handed over full control to him. Cookworthy had been patient and enduring, coaxing them when they needed coaxing, tolerating their temperamental moments but always getting the best out of them through careful management. Of the two, Thibault was the most difficult to handle, but Henri Saqui was also very volatile and voluble. He was liable to moods, at times being prepared to work late into the night on a piece and at other times grudging every hour spent in what he considered an execrable climate. Champion was

69

everything that Cookworthy was not—he was young, headstrong, impetuous and impetuous, and as such he was not the man to deal with Gallic temperaments.

Cookworthy remained associated with the Bristol porcelain works for two years. He did not spend all the time at Bristol, but travelled backwards and forwards, no easy task in those days of primitive roads and poor transport. Most of his time at Bristol was spent in pacifying Thibault and Saqui, both of whom threatened they would not stay an instant if he were no longer in charge. Some good pieces were produced at Bristol during this period, including some rather beautiful vases, chimney-piece garnitures and table centre-pieces in the forms of shells such as cockles, clams and scallops. The white porcelain produced at Bristol showed that by this time, Cookworthy had more fully mastered the techniques of firing his pieces. There are fewer firing defects such as specking, peppering and fire-cracking, and smoke staining was much less prevalent. At Plymouth, such cups as had been produced, were straight sided coffee cups of simple design, and saucers were really shallow dishes, but at Bristol, the technique of making cups and saucers was mastered, and so more of them were produced. The shapes of the cups were altered also, some being fluted and moulded and others having delicately curved sides. Dishes were produced in a greater variety, but were still not entirely successful. The decoration of these pieces was mostly either rococo, with swags, scrolls, flourishes and garlands liberally distributed, or pseudo-Chinese with supposed Oriental trees, flowers and birds. Saqui was the rococo expert, but both Bone and Stephens had become quite adept at imitating his workmanship by this time.

In 1774, Cookworthy decided that he had experienced enough of travelling backwards and forwards to Bristol, and therefore assigned his patent over to Richard Champion. The terms under which this was achieved were that the latter should pay Cookworthy or his heirs so much each year for the use of the patent. The draft read as follows:

"I, William Cookworthy, chemist of Plymouth, in the County of Devon, do hereby assign my portion of that patent, entitled "Manufacture of Porcelain" to Richard Champion gentleman of Castle Green in the city of Bristol,

on the conditions that he shall pay to me, my executors or
assignees a sum annually equivalent to that which he shall
pay to Mr. Pitt for rent, dues etc."

The amount paid by Champion to Cookworthy annually from
1774-1778, was about £120. Champion found that this agree-
ment, coming as it did on top of all his other financial commitments, was very burdensome. Before he could produce a single
piece of porcelain, he had to pay rent for the pit to Thomas Pitt,
together with so many shillings per ton of clay or stone produced, in addition to which he had to pay the cost of trans-
porting the clay and stone to Bristol and pay the Cookworthys
their share as well. This put the final price of his porcelain out of
the reach of all but the most wealthy, and as a result, with the
decline in trade his financial resources became very strained. He
did, however, succeed in carrying on until 1778.

As might have been expected, immediately Champion
assumed full control of the Bristol porcelain factory, Saqui and
Thibault tendered their resignations. What happened to Saqui
after this is not known. It is doubtful whether he would have
returned to France, in view of the political situation there, and it
is possible that he may either have gone into retirement or gone
to work for another concern. Thibault went straight over to
Wedgwood, who found him to be absolutely infuriating. "Our
new modeller would have made a shocking ugly thing of the
lamp if he had been left to himself" was one of Wedgwood's
comments, although it is true this may have been due to a change
in fashion making Thibault's mouldings seem old fashioned and
outmoded. The modeller only stayed at Etruria for a year, and
after he had left, Wedgwood's remaining modellers tried to
charge him double for their work, because it was cheaper than
"Mr. Tebo's", his work hardly ever having been properly
finished.

Champion's production would have ground to a halt sooner
than 1778, had he not had some patrons who placed substantial
orders with him. A number of influential and wealthy Bristol
families placed orders for tea services, and these orders helped keep
him going. He found that in order to gain this custom he had to
change the style of his decoration. This was the period when the
rococo and Oriental type decorations began to go out of fashion,

being replaced with the late eighteenth century neo-classicism, as typified in the work of Adam and his contemporaries. The styles used by the porcelain factories of Meissen, Vienna and Dresden a decade or so before were also beginning to catch on at this time, and Champion produced some pieces which were definitely Meissenesque. From Champion's productions during this period, it would seem that he also subscribed to Cookworthy's earlier belief that porcelain "should be both of use and beauty", as the bulk of his work was quality porcelain for use in the home. Like Cookworthy, he made teapots, coffee pots, sauce boats and jugs, but the latter were somewhat different in design to those made at Plymouth. His pieces also included chocolate pots and chocolate cups in the German style—chocolate as a beverage having just caught on—and some massive moulded tureens and tureen stands. Cookworthy's efforts at gilding had never been very successful. He had found difficulty in making the gilding stick, and even when it did, it seldom was absolutely true in colour, often having a greenish to greyish tinge. Champion's gilding was much better, looking really like what gold should do. Amongst his commissions were several services for various guilds and professional bodies, and some really fine services decorated with family coats of arms, crests and monograms. One of the most elaborate was the service especially designed by him for his friend and patron Edmund Burke, the great Radical member for Bristol.

In 1775, Champion applied for an extension of the Cookworthy patent for a further fourteen years. When the application was laid before Parliament, Wedgwood and Turner of Lane End, both of whom were anxious to get their hands legally on supplies of china clay, lobbied Parliamentary opposition to it. So vigorous was their campaign, that in the end, all Champion was left with was a very much mutilated version of the original patent, giving him very little protection compared with what had been accorded Cookworthy by his original patent. The costs of defending his case, on top of all his other commitments left him so financially embarrassed that he could no longer carry on the factory, by 1778, being virtually out of production. For the next two years, the kilns were only fired sporadically to produce a few special orders. He was looking around for someone to whom he could transfer the 99-year lease of Carloggas and the Pitt-Cookworthy dues. Finally, in December 1780, he formed a company made up of eight potters, and this company bought the patent from him. They began once again manufacturing hand porcelain to the Cookworthy formula, slightly modified. The eight potters involved were John Turner of Lane End, Anthony Keeling, Charles Bagnall, Samual Hollins, Jacob Warburton, William Clowes, Joshua Heath and John Daniel. Shortly after the formation of the company, originally known as Hollins, Warburton, Daniel & Co., Turner and Keeling withdrew, leaving the other six to carry on. The company later became known as the New Hall Company of Shelton, taking its name from Shelton in Staffordshire.

In 1782 Champion withdrew from the New Hall Company, thus severing the last links between it and the Quaker potting fraternity. His friend Edmund Burke, a member of the Rockingham administration, offered him the post of Paymaster General of His Majesty's Forces. Two years later, when the government was ousted by the Tories, he emigrated to South Carolina, where he died in 1791 at the age of 48, having only survived his old friend Cookworthy by eleven years.

VIII. THE DECLINING YEARS

WHEN COOKWORTHY FINALLY RELINQUISHED HIS HOLD over the Bristol Porcelain Factory in 1774, he was a very tired man. Although then only sixty-nine, he had put so much into life that physically he was a much older man. All he wished to do was to concentrate on his Quaker Ministry during his declining years, leaving the world of commerce to younger and fitter men. In his heyday he had been slim, straight and tall, now he had grown stooped and somewhat portly, but there was still the same gentle manner and kindly smile that had endeared him to so many people during the previous sixty odd years. He could no longer get around as well as he had formerly done, having become somewhat rheumatic. As he confided to a friend: "I must confess that at times I feel a great weariness which descends upon me like a great weight. I have to carry it around as a burden, which at times is hard to bear. However, I know that I must do that which the Lord doth require of me ere my time shall come, and if I have not strength, He has strength to help me through."

After 1774, he travelled but little, apart from going to the Quaker meetings at nearby Bretonside. This he would never neglect, no matter how weary he felt before he went. He used to say "I go into the Lord's house weary and worn, ravelled with the cares of age and time, but in His house, I find a great peace which brings new strength to me, and I go out a younger man in spirit than when I came." He was always at home to any of his old friends amongst the Naval officers and merchantmen, who appreciated his conversation, for his declining health had brought no diminution of his mental powers. He had the capacity, not always present with great talkers, of being able also to be a sympathetic listener, and he could always be relied upon for some sound advice.

At this late stage in life, he became more and more interested in the Swedenborgian philosophy, and would debate it with a vigour which would have done credit to a much younger man. There were those who, previously unable to understand the Swedenborgian viewpoint, would find after a discussion with Cookworthy, that it had all become clearer in their minds. Cookworthy had, of course, developed a form of natural philosophy of his own. In his life, he had seen moments of great sadness, sadness so deep that it had seemed impossible to bear, but also he had had moments of great elation, such as the time when he first beheld his first born Lydia cradled in her mother's arms, and when he first beheld the "caulin" in the workings of Wheal Grey on Tregonning Hill. He had been a friend of famous men, like Captain Cook and Sir Joshua Reynolds, and he had been a friend of humble men, like Daniel Gumb of The Cheesewring and Richard Yelland, the farmer at Carloggas, and throughout all his experiences, his encounters and his friendships he felt the working of the hand of God. He never went back to Cockside in sadness to ponder on what might have been, but accepted what life had brought him, embodying it in the text from Philippians 4.11 "I have learned, in whatsoever state I am, therewith to be content."

In 1775, when he heard of the trouble that his friend Richard Champion was undergoing in trying to renew his patent, his heart was sad, knowing the nature of the opposition. "Poor Richard is like a lamb, facing the lions. I pray that the Lord will give him courage to endure." He himself wanted no more to do with it personally. "What I had to do, that I did, but now, if the Lord wills, I shall have had done with it." Aged as he was, he did not relish the idea of having to do battle against such formidable opponents as Josiah Wedgwood I, John Turner, and Thomas Bentley. He had always been a man of peace, and had never wanted any business he had undertaken to be a cause of strife. He believed in the adage, "Where there is commerce, there is conflict". People have criticized him for trying to keep his discovery a secret, and have accused him of being selfish. Certainly his discovery was not widely talked about, until he was ready to announce his invention to the world, but this was not of his designing, specifically. Many people in Cornwall knew of what he was doing, and he himself made no secret of his actions. He came and went openly, discussing his aims and ambitions with people like John Nancarrow, Dr. Hingston, Thomas Pitt, James

Fox and many others. His shipments of clay and stone were made quite openly from Polmear (now known as Charlestown) and were unloaded at Cockside Wharf in full view of anyone who wanted to see. Everyone in Cockside knew what was going on, and there was considerable excitement when word got round that he had at last perfected his process for the production of porcelain. Although the nucleus of his staff was drawn from Bow, he also employed many local persons during the time that his factory was in operation, and no one was sworn to secrecy. This was in complete contrast to what had happened in Saxony, where Bottger, having discovered a method of producing a type of hard porcelain, was kept virtually a prisoner by Friedrich Augustus unless the secret should leak out.

In 1776, the family had another of its times of great sadness when Philip Cookworthy died. He was only 60 years old. The most travelled of all the Cookworthys, he had made numerous voyages to the Far East as a boy and had served his elder brother faithfully all the years he had spent at the pharmacy, taking complete charge of it after 1755, when Cookworthy was at his busiest experimenting with the porcelain. With Philip's death, the management of the pharmacy passed to Benjamin, the youngest of the brothers, then 58 years of age. He had worked all his life in the pharmacy, so that it was only fit and proper that he should at last get the chance to take charge of it himself.

Another event in the life of the Cookworthys in 1776 was the last visit they were to receive from Captain James Cook, that courageous Yorkshireman who had found a way into the hearts of all of them over the years. Cook found Cookworthy much aged in body, but not a whit less active in spirit. His mind was as sharp as ever, and he bombarded the explorer with numerous questions concerning voyages in the past and the voyage he was about to undertake. At their parting, Cookworthy felt a sadness greater than ever before. Whether he had a premonition of impending disaster is not known, but he grasped Cook by the hand and said, "Take care brother, take great care. Our thoughts are with thee. May God go with thee wherever thou goest, and may He bless thee in all thy undertakings".

When Cook left Plymouth, he went by way of Good Hope, south of Tasmania to New Zealand, then on to the Society

Islands and Hawaii. From there he explored the West Coast of America as far as the Bering Straits before returning to Hawaii, where he was killed by the natives in 1779. Cookworthy's feelings on parting had been right—he was not to see his brave and venturous friend again. He had known Cook since he was first promoted to the rank of captain, many years before.

In 1777, something happened to gladden the hearts of all the Cookworthys. Susanna, or Sukey as she was called, who had been courted by a Quaker from London, George Harrison, finally married him. She was 34 years old and her husband was 30. She was destined to be luckier in marriage than either of her two sisters in that she would not lose her husband early. In fact, he eventually outlived her by seventeen years, but the whole of their 33 years of married life together were very happy. She was to have by him three daughters, Lydia, Susanna and Mary, before having her only son, George, who was born so late in her life that she had practically given up hoping for any further family, being then 47 years of age. Sukey was her father's favourite, as much as any child can be a favourite in a Quaker household, and he was greatly pleased that she had at last married. It had been thought that perhaps she, like her eldest sister Lydia, might stay unmarried. Cookworthy was rather restricted in his movements and infirm by this time, and spent a great deal of his time sitting in front of the fire reading. It was almost in the last year of his life that he finally consented to sit for a portrait. His friend, Dr. John Wolcot, better known as the satirist Peter Pindar, had acquired a protégé, a young painter from Cornwall called John Opie. This lad had shown a natural aptitude for portraiture, and had already produced several portraits before undertaking one of Cookworthy. When he did the painting he was nineteen years of age and Cookworthy was 74. The picture, although lacking the polish of Opie's later portraits, was nevertheless said to be a good likeness. He painted exactly what he saw, a kindly old man, drawing near to the time that he should meet his Maker, but with a mind still active and alert.*

---

* The picture may be seen to this day, in the Plymouth City Museum, the same place where so much of his finest porcelain is housed.

Cookworthy began to fail rapidly in 1780, and his family were aware that the end was near. Sometimes he was obviously drifting very close to the borderline between the here and the hereafter, and could on occasions be heard murmuring gently as if to someone unseen but felt. His family heard the name Sarah on his lips on more than one occasion, and knew that he was drawing close in spirit to his dear wife, who had been taken from him 35 years before. As summer gave way to autumn he seemed for a while to rally, and talked more with his relatives and friends, but this was like the setting sun, which sometimes sends a last bright gleam across the sky before sinking below the horizon. On October 17th, he died peacefully, with members of his family and friends close beside him. He himself had been fully aware of his impending death, being calmly resigned to it. His friend and kinswoman Lydia Fox visited him just before his death, and wrote: "His senses remained perfectly clear throughout the whole of the last weeks. He told a friend whom he loved that he found himself troubled with the pangs of approaching death, knowing however that these must soon pass. He was satisfied that nothing less than a miracle could restore him, but was under no apprehension concerning the same. He said that he experienced much calmness and resignation, having been supported through the present trial for the comfort of grief of his approaching happiness."

His lifelong friend James Fox who was present at his death, described it as follows:

"He continued to grow weaker, and his voice was so much altered that it was difficult to understand him, but his senses remained unimpaired, and his surrounding friends had the satisfaction of seeing him in possession of that peace of mind which supported him a great deal in calmness through the trial, giving him an unshaken confidence of his approaching happiness. At last, our beloved relation was removed from the church militant to the church triumphant. He died this morning soon after 7 o'clock without sigh or breath. I was at the bedside at the time, but could not distinguish the instant he quitted mortality. He retained his senses to the last moment, so I believe, though he could not speak for many hours before his departure. We shall most sensibly feel his loss, but be thankful that he was favoured with such full assurance of entering into bliss. I humbly hope that many of us who were witnesses of his happy state, will bear it in remembrance, to encourage us to pursue that sense of conduct which will ensure the favour of him."

James Fox was also present at the funeral, which he described as follows:

"The last first day, (Sunday) the remains of our dear friend were removed from his house about 2.0 o'c in the afternoon, the number of people who attended at the door being many and there being a large addition made as the corpse passed along. There were hundreds more at the meeting house than it could contain, and some had much difficulty in getting in. Eventually, however, after some little time had elapsed, the people were still, and Thomas Pole prayed for the soul of our dear brother. He was followed by T. Binnes in prayer and then he (Thos. Pole) preached the sermon. Towards the latter part of this service, he spoke of the deceased very properly saying "Notwithstanding his amazing capacious understanding, he possessed that state of a little child". The text for the sermon was taken from "Except a man be born again, he cannot enter the Kingdom of Heaven". Cookworthy was interred in the burial ground belonging to the Society of Friends at Treville Street, Bretonside, behind the Meeting House. His remains were there until the site was purchased by the Corporation for the purposes of clearance, when they were transferred, together with the remains of all the other Quakers to the Plymouth Corporation Cemetery at Efford.

The following obituary was printed in a provincial newspaper circulating the Plymouth area, dated October 20th 1780. "Last Tuesday morning died Mr. William Cookworthy of Plymouth, an eminent minister of the people called Quakers, and one of the greatest chemists this nation ever produced. With strong natural talents sanctified by the religion of his divine maker, full of love and goodwill for all mankind, he practically recommended the universal principle which influenced his whole conduct. Since simplicity and wisdom were heavily united in his character, the goodness of his heart, the greatness of his understanding, the persuasiveness of his manner and his universal knowledge rendered his company and conversation useful, interesting and pleasing. A philosopher without pride, a Christian without bigotry, he lived beloved by all for the faith of his friendship, and after a life dedicated to the service of Christianity with a stake in confidence in his approaching felicity, having fought the good fight of faith, he laid hold of eternal life through Jesus Christ his Saviour, being favoured while here with an undoubted evidence that he should be admitted into that Kingdom into which the Saints and Knights rejoice evermore."

His family received a number of messages from members of the naval fraternity, with whom he had had many years of association. One captain said: "I feel the loss of a true friend, one of the kind whose friendship will endure down the years and be extinguished only by death. Whenever I put into port, I would make my way to Notte Street, and there I would be assured of a warm welcome. He was always eager to hear tales I had to tell of far away places, places that I feel he would have loved to have visited, himself had he had the opportunity. I could always rely on him to give me a fair account of all that had happened during my absence, and to give me a straight appraisal of all affairs of State both at home and in the Colonies." This gives an insight into his contacts with seafaring men. In the days when there were no means of mass communication, and there were no methods for getting news out to ships at sea, captains undertaking long voyages would be out of touch with the situations at home from the time they left until the time that they returned. Governments could rise and governments could fall; taxes be imposed or taxes repealed; new laws could be passed and old ones done away with, and they would not know about any of it. So it was, that on reaching port they would repair to that quiet old Quaker, William Cookworthy, who would tell them all they needed to know, he himself always keeping abreast of the situations both at home and abroad.

Cookworthy's family, although they did not express themselves in the same way as these outside contacts, nevertheless missed their father greatly. No matter what he had been involved in, whether it was the work of the pharmacy, or long time-consuming experiments, he would still always find time to listen to them. In times of bereavement, as his two widowed daughters would avow, he was always ready to offer spiritual consolation, and when he was himself bereaved, he would endure it with great courage, so as not to let his grief impinge on others or affect them in any way. His family knew, however, that this show of courage was not due to lack of feeling. He had deep feelings, but would always keep them inwardly. As he himself said: "My feelings are kept between my heart and myself".

Tributes were even paid to him by people who normally had little time for the Quakers and what they stood for. An example of this was a testimonial from someone with whom he had regularly done business at Notte Street: "There has passed an honest man. In all the years that I dealt with him, he was always scrupulously fair in all his negotiations. He neither exacted more than his due, nor paid more than was his due. He would ask a fair price and pay a fair price, and he would only deal with honest merchants. Those who were dealing in plundered goods, obtained through the fortunes of war by diverse means, he would not deal with, regarding their wares as ill-gotten gains. Also, if anyone showed him dishonesty or false dealing, he would have none of him after."

Cookworthy himself never lost his natural humility, and in his last years, anyone seeing him, not knowing his past, would have never credited him with being a great discoverer. His own summary of his achievements was characteristic of him: "God placed on me a great responsibility, when He led me to the true china earth. It was that I should strive by all my means of human endeavour to unfold the secret of the making of the true porcelain ware, and that I should then declare that discovery to all mankind. Of myself, I achieved nothing. What was accomplished, God accomplished through me. He bade me ask, and I received, He bade me seek and I found."

IX. THE LATER COOKWORTHYS

COOKWORTHY'S ONLY SADNESS WAS THAT HE SHOULD have no son to succeed him, although his daughters were all very dear to him, and he made as adequate provisions for all of them after his death as his means would allow, through shares in the pharmacy and such income as was coming in from the use of his patent. Of his own brothers, Philip had predeceased him, but Benjamin lived until 1785, dying at the age of 67, and Jacob, the longest lived of all the family, lived until 1796, when he was 87 years old. Benjamin managed the pharmacy up to the time of his death, after which it passed into the hands of Francis Fox, Cookworthy's grandson by his daughter Sarah.

Cookworthy's daughters never matched their uncle Jacob for longevity. Lydia, who never married, but looked after her father in his latter years, died in 1791 at the age of 55. Sarah Fox outlived her husband by 48 years, finally dying in 1814 at the age of 76. Mary, widowed early, like herself, died in 1809 at the age of 69, and Sukey (Susannah Harrison), who had the happiest married life of all of them, died in 1810 at the age of 67. Only Sarah and Susanna were survived by any heirs. Sarah's son William Fox changed his name by deed poll to William Fox Cookworthy, and married twice. His first wife was Tabitha Fox, a distant cousin, daughter of Edward Fox of Wadebridge and Anna Were, daughter of the Thomas Were who was married to the sister of Sarah Berry Cookworthy, and who had been a shareholder in the Plymouth Porcelain Factory. On her death, he married Elizabeth Howard, but neither of his wives bore him any children. Apart from William, Sarah Fox also had a daughter Sarah Fox who died unmarried, and a son Francis Fox. It was this son who carried on the Notte Street Pharmacy after the death of Benjamin Cookworthy. Francis married Sarah Birkbeck, daughter of John Birkbeck of Settle in Yorkshire and had two children, Francis who died in infancy, and Sarah, who married William Dillworth Crewdson of Kendal. Francis himself died in 1812.

Susannah Harrison had four children in all, three girls and one boy. Her first, Lydia, born in 1779, married twice, the first husband being Richard Shepley and the second her cousin Thomas Harrison, son of George Harrison's brother William. Susannah's second child was called Susanna after her mother. She was born in 1780 and died at the age of eight in 1788. The third daughter was Mary, born in 1782, after which there was a gap of eight years before the birth of her only son, George, when she was 47 years old. George, although rather unexpected, was nevertheless welcome. He became a barrister when he grew up, and wrote a life of William Cookworthy. He married Mary Coleman in 1823, and by her had three daughters and a son, the same as his mother. The daughters were called Elizabeth, Jane and Lydia, the son being called William Cookworthy Harrison. Jane and Lydia both died in infancy from the same infection in 1836, one being then four and the other six. William died in America, without issue. Elizabeth married Theodore Compton, who also wrote a life of Cookworthy. Such descendants of Cookworthy's who are alive today are descended from the fruits of this union.

Several of the Compton family have distinguished themselves in one way or another. Elizabeth Compton's son Edward Theodore Compton became a well known landscape painter. Of his sons, Alwyn Theodore Compton F.R.C.S. was a highly respected surgeon, who died in 1942. Alwyn's brother Edward married Gertrude Dietsch, and his youngest brother, William Cookworthy Compton M.A., became headmaster of Dover College. He died in 1936 at the age of 82. Of his two children, Ethelwyn married Francis Duckworth C.B.E., and her brother Cuthred Compton B.A., married Sophia Hope Gorham.

The known survivors of William Cookworthy, today, are all descended from the landscape artist E. T. Compton. He married a German girl, Auguste Plotz in 1872, and apart from his sons Alwyn, Edward and William, also had two daughters, Dora and Margaret. Dora married Frederick Keel, and by him had two daughters, Mary and Barbara and a son, Frederick Compton Keel, born in 1913. He duly married one Pauline Gundy and had two children, John Christopher Keel and Philippa Keel, who, it is believed are both still alive. Margaret Compton married a surgeon, James Cole Marshall, F.R.C.S., by whom she had two daughters, Margaret Elfrida and Ruth. Margaret Elfrida Marshall married Edward Danson Steel, and their family, as far as is known, all survive. Peter Danson Steel and his brother Bernard Alwyn Steel both live in Streatham, London, S.W.16. Apart from these, there are thought to be some descendants bearing the name Harrison, being descended from the Lydia Harrison whose second husband was her cousin Thomas Harrison. They are said to have had sons and grandsons, some of whose progeny are probably still alive, although their exact whereabouts are not known.

The Notte Street Pharmacy, established by Cookworthy in 1725, was closed down in 1812 on the death of Francis Fox. It was reopened directly in new premises under the management of Benjamin Balkwill, who had worked with Fox at Notte Street. Balkwill managed the business jointly with Joseph Cookworthy, Benjamin's son and William Charles Prideaux, grandson of Philip Cookworthy. The new premises were in Whimple Street, but the business did not remain there very long before being moved yet again, this time to 106 Old Town Street, where it traded as Balkwill's, formerly Cookworthy & Bevan. Balkwill is thought to have been some distant connection of the Cookworthys, his family being Quakers from the Aveton Gifford and Loddiswell areas close to Kingsbridge. He himself had married a distant relative of the Cookworthy brothers, Elizabeth Hancock, whose great-grandparents were Robert and Mary Debell of Looe, (Cookworthy's grandparents), in the year 1800. It has been said of the Cornish Quakers that all were cousins, and it appears that this also applied to the Devonshire Quakers.

When Joseph Cookworthy died, his interest in the Old Town Street Pharmacy passed to his son, Joseph Collin Cookworthy, but as he was busy with his practice as a physician and surgeon, he left the running of the business to Benjamin Balkwill. Dr. Cookworthy was then nearly forty years of age. The business remained at 106 Old Town Street under the management of successive members of the Balkwill family until the retirement of A. P. Balkwill before the war. During the bombing of Plymouth by the Luftwaffe, the Old Town Street Pharmacy was completely destroyed, which was a great tragedy, as it was a lovely old Georgian building, well worthy of preservation. It was a tragedy also, for another reason. Not only did it still have the traditional atmosphere of an old established pharmacy, such as must have been familiar to Cookworthy himself, but it also possessed some drug jars which were originally owned by Cookworthy and had been handled by him. In addition, preserved in a glass case, as an object of some reverence, was a beautiful blue porcelain drug jar, said to be the first piece of Cookworthy blue ware ever made, after he had learned the secret of making blue from zaffre (cobalt blue) from Roger Keniston of Bristol. Keniston used imported zaffre, ground down with mortar and slab, but Cookworthy subsequently made use of Cornish flowers of cobalt, roasting it to drive off the arsenic content. All the Cookworthy drug jars were destroyed in the bombing. After this date, the pharmacy continued in temporary premises until the rebuilding of Plymouth City Centre, when it was rehoused at permanent premises in Cornwall Street, and still trades as Balkwill & Co. (Chemists) Ltd.

The manufacture of hard porcelain, begun by Cookworthy and continued by Richard Champion, was carried on subsequently by the New Hall Company of Shelton, until about 1810, after which the Company went over to making bone china. Practically no hard porcelain is now made commercially in Britain, since public taste, after the introduction of bone china by Josiah Spode, created a demand for that type of soft paste porcelain rather than for the hard paste Oriental type ware. Soft paste, however, has never been as durable as hard paste, as was borne out during the war, when the Plymouth Athenaeum was burnt down as a result of incendiary bombs. The articles made of Cookworthy's hard paste survived the fire, even if they were blackened by smoke, bearing out the claim he made that "our ware doth withstand heat and the fire, being equal in this respect to the Asiatic ware". At the Athenaeum there were two white porcelain pheasants. Both of these had been damaged prior to 1939 and had lost their tails. The tails were replaced, but in soft paste, not in hard paste. In the great heat of the conflagration, the soft paste replacement tails melted away, whilst the original Cookworthy white porcelain survived intact. No one expected, when the ruins of the buildings were excavated, to find any of the porcelain intact, but it was. No fitter testimonial than this could be found for the claims Cookworthy had made.

X. TWO HUNDRED YEARS AFTER

THE PRESENT DAY STUDENT, SEEKING TO VISIT THE PLACES known and loved by Cookworthy, will find many of them difficult to discover and others that would not be recognisable to Cookworthy, were he to visit them. Two hundred years is a long time, buildings have decayed and have been pulled down, buildings have been bombed and demolished, and many places are no longer known by the same names as they were two centuries ago. There are, however, some places which can be visited. In Kingsbridge, the old grammar school still stands, converted into a William Cookworthy Memorial Museum with the aid of English China Clays Ltd. There is some doubt as to whereabouts in Kingsbridge he lived, some authorities saying that in fact he lived just outside the town in one of the surrounding villages. Kingsbridge itself, however, still has some of the buildings apart from the school which he must have seen and known.

In Plymouth, bombing has obliterated many of the places associated with him, whilst rebuilding has destroyed others. Notte Street and Old Town Street still exist as names, although the latter was very severely bombed and subsequently rebuilt. His pharmacy in Notte Street is said to have stood on the site where the Elim Church now stands. The old Friends Meeting House and the burial ground behind it at Bretonside are no more, their place having been taken by the Bretonside developments. The Society of Friends now meet at Swarthmore in Mutley Plain, but still preserve some of the old records, however. The mortal remains of the Friends, apart from Cookworthy himself, are buried in a common grave at Efford Cemetery, and this must include all the members of his family who were originally interred at the Treville Street burial ground—his mother, his wife, his brothers and sisters and his daughters. Cockside, now known as Coxside, must look rather different to what it did in his day. The wharf remains, but the buildings on it have changed.

87

There is no trace of his cloam kiln, and his other establishment at Cockside is said to have been where the Plymouth Corporation Gasworks now stands.

In the Godolphin area, in Cornwall, one can still see the remains of the workings of Wheal Grey, on Tregonning Hill as well as the china stone quarries at Hensafraen, and one can also see the remains of the Great Work mine where he saw china clay in use. Where John Nancarrow actually lived, however, is not certain. At Fowey, there is now no trace of the bell foundry, which must have ceased to exist as far back as the late 18th century, after which bells were sent away from Fowey to be founded. It has been suggested that the building may have been a general foundry, which just cast bells as part of its operations. One can still see china stone, used as a building material in the towers of St. Columb and St. Stephen parish churches, as Cookworthy saw it.

At St. Stephen, there is still a Carloggas Farm, although it is doubtful whether its present appearance is exactly as it was at the time when Richard Yelland was the tenant there. The remains of Cookworthy's earliest pits at Rescrowsa and Carloggas are still to be seen, although some scrambling through undergrowth in places is necessary. His later pit on Trethosa Moor has long since been replaced by a gigantic gaping hole, one half of which is worked by E.C.L.P. as Trethosa Pit, and the other half by the Goonvean Company as Goonvean pit. This is the deepest, and in the Trethosa section, the oldest clay pit still in production.

The white scar on the hillside of King Pippins Mount (St. Stephen's Beacon) has long since become grassed over. The opencast and costeaning operations carried out in Cookworthy's time, when the workings were known as the Carloggas Mine, were later abandoned in favour of shaft mining. The working became known as Tinhill Mine, although little tin was extracted from it. The remains of the old engine-house, now sadly dilapidated, are still just visible above the undergrowth. The view from the Beacon, however, has drastically changed since the time of Cookworthy. In his day, all one would have seen from it would have been other bleak hillsides, some covered with coarse grass or heather, others with furze, hawthorn or blackthorn. Today, these uplands have been replaced by numerous gaping chasms, each accompanied by its shining white pyramid of sand, known variously as sand bu.rows, sandtips and skytips. These are not eyesores in the ways that most slagheaps and spoiltips are, but blend into the landscape, making the terrain have, from the distance, the appearance of a mountain range similar to the Spanish and South American Sierras.

The extraction of clay and stone, which in the lifetime of Cookworthy was confined to a small area including Trethosa, Rescrowsa, Treviscoe, St. Dennis and Carloggas, now extends over a much larger area, taking in Whitemoor, Nanpean, Roche and Bugle, and even extending as far as the outer environs of St. Blazey. China clay is also extracted on Bodmin Moor, at Stannon Marsh, Hawks' Tor and Parsons Park, also from several pits on the south-western edge of Dartmoor, including Cholwichtown, Lee Moor, Shaugh Lake and Whitehill. Every pit and every tip which exists today, does so as a monument to the man who first had the insight to recognise china clay for what it was, William Cookworthy, the Porcelain Man, who might almost also have been called the first China Clay Man.

SOURCES

The information in the preceding pages has been drawn from a great variety of sources. These include the biographies of Cookworthy produced by George Harrison, his grandson, Theodore Compton, his great-grand-daughter's husband and John Prideaux, the great-grandson of his brother Philip. Other sources have included the Fox-Hingston letters and sundry other documents. The Society of Friends have provided some very useful items of information otherwise unobtainable.

The author wishes to acknowledge his gratitude to W. H. Wingate, F.B.O.A., for his assistance in providing a precise genealogical tree for the Cookworthy family which was of very great assistance in carrying out the research.

INDEX